Health Benefits of Curcumin

Edited by Santosh K. Kar

Published in London, United Kingdom

Health Benefits of Curcumin
http://dx.doi.org/10.5772/intechopen.1007218
Edited by Santosh K. Kar

Contributors
Dini Kesuma, Farida Anwari, Galih Satrio Putra, Kirti S. Pawar, Lubiao Liang, Melanny Ika Sulistyowaty, Muhammad Ainur Hasan, Rajnandini S. Pawar, Samragni S. Pawar, Santosh K. Kar, Satheesh K. Pawar, Shimaa E. Rashad, Sitabja Mukherjee, Yajin Zhao

First published in London, United Kingdom, 2025 by IntechOpen
IntechOpen is the global imprint of INTECHOPEN LIMITED, registered in England and Wales, registration number: 11086078, 167-169 Great Portland Street, London, W1W 5PF, United Kingdom

For EU product safety concerns: IN TECH d.o.o., Prolaz Marije Krucifikse Kozulić 3, 51000 Rijeka, Croatia, info@intechopen.com or visit our website at intechopen.com.

British Library Cataloguing-in-Publication Data
A catalogue record for this book is available from the British Library

Health Benefits of Curcumin
Edited by Santosh K. Kar
p. cm.
Print ISBN 978-1-83635-001-9
Online ISBN 978-1-83635-000-2
eBook (PDF) ISBN 978-1-83635-002-6

Meet the editor

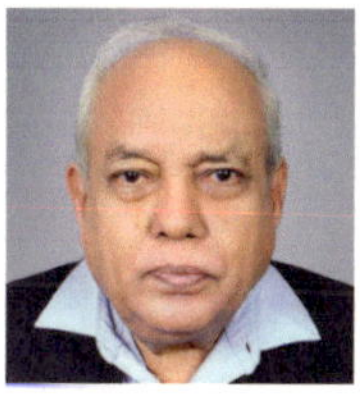

Prof. Santosh Kar is an Immunology Teacher with research experience in Filariasis, Malaria and Tuberculosis. Founder Director of ICMR's Regional Medical Research Centre at Bhubaneswar and Chairman of Centre for Biotechnology at Jawaharlal Nehru University, New Delhi, and holds a patent on Nano Curcumin.

Contents

Preface

With an increase in life expectancy, people are living longer and have to cope with a greater incidence of chronic and age-related diseases arising out of chronic inflammation and immune dysfunction, like Heart disease, Alzheimer's disease, Diabetes, Osteoarthritis and Cancer. These diseases can significantly impact quality of life. Therefore, how to age while remaining healthy is a matter of great concern. Polyphenols, the naturally occurring compounds abundant in fruits, vegetables, and spices, have emerged as promising agents for promoting healthy ageing by combating oxidative stress, inflammation, and immune malfunction, which are the key drivers of age-related pathologies.

Among the polyphenols, curcumin, derived from the rhizome of the *Curcuma longa* plant, stands out for its antioxidant, anti-inflammatory, and antimicrobial properties. Its unique chemical structure, coupled with its favourable safety profile, has spurred extensive research into its chemical and pharmacological properties. This book explores these aspects in detail, beginning with an in-depth analysis of curcumin's molecular characteristics and their implications for clinical use.

After the introductory chapter, the second chapter of this book, "Chemical and Physical Properties, Pharmacokinetics, and Pharmacodynamics of Curcumin Derivatives", describes all these aspects very lucidly.

Most Viral infections are zoonotic, meaning they infect humans when they cross the human-animal barrier and become virulent. When such infections become pandemic-like, as the recent COVID-19 pandemic has, and kill human beings in large numbers, control becomes an urgent necessity. As vaccine development or the creation of specific antiviral drugs takes time, natural compounds like curcumin become a promising adjunct therapy. Preclinical studies have shown that curcumin inhibits SARS-CoV-2 virus infection, controls cytokine storm induced by it and reduces lung injury and fibrosis. This has been described in the third chapter of this book, "Role of Curcumin to Prevent (Thrombotic) Complications of Viral (COVID) Infections".

While curcumin's antiviral properties highlight its potential in acute infectious diseases, its neuroprotective capabilities extend its therapeutic reach to chronic conditions, such as Parkinson's disease (PD), Alzheimer's disease (AD), and multiple sclerosis (MS). To target it specifically to brain cells and break the aggregation of amyloid β-sheet conformations, curcumin nanoparticles have been functionalized with brain-specific ligands, which would facilitate their delivery into the brain. This has been described in the fourth chapter of this book, "Potential Clinical Value of Curcumin and Its Therapeutic Benefits in Cancer and Human Health".

Curcumin can modulate multiple molecular targets which are involved in cancer development and progression. It exerts its anticancer effects by inactivating various signalling pathways, including the suppression of NF-κB, JAK/STAT3, and PI3K/Akt, as well as the modulation of cell cycle regulators. It has been demonstrated that third-generation formulations, composed of pure natural curcumin with natural emulsifiers, when combined with innovative drug delivery systems, such as nanoparticles or liposomes, can treat patients more effectively. This has been elaborated in the 5th chapter of this book, "Curcumin in Cancer Therapy: Mechanisms, Delivery Systems, and Clinical Potential".

The interplay between curcumin, gut microbiota, and tumor microenvironments presents new opportunities for personalized cancer therapy. By leveraging gut microbiota metabolites to enhance curcumin's efficacy, even at low bioavailability, and disrupting the immunosuppressive environments within the tumor microbiome, researchers aim to optimize the therapeutic outcomes of curcumin-based treatment formulations. This concept is explained in Chapter 6 of the book "Nanocurcumin Formulations for Immunotherapy of Cancer".

The unstinting support of Ms. Mia Vulovic, Publishing Process Manager at IntechOpen, to the Academic Editor—not only during the writing of my chapter but also throughout the review of submitted chapters and their compilation into book form—is gratefully acknowledged. Without her guidance and help, the book could not have been completed.

Santosh K. Kar
Polyfeenolix Research Laboratory,
Biotechnology Incubator,
KIIT University,
Bhubaneswar, Odisha, India

Chapter 1

Introductory Chapter: Health Benefits of Curcumin

Santosh K. Kar

1. Introduction

Curcumin (1,7-bis(4-hydroxy-3-methoxyphenol)-1,6-heptadiene-3,5-dione) belongs to the curcuminoid class of molecules, which is present in the rhizome of a *Curcuma longa* plant, which gives turmeric its medicinal properties. It has two aromatic rings containing o-methoxy phenolic groups, which are connected by a seven carbon linker containing an α,β-unsaturated β-diketone group. This unique structure enables curcumin to remain in keto-enol tautomeric form depending upon the pH of the milieu in which it exists and exhibit hydrogen donation reactions leading to oxidation of curcumin, or reversible and irreversible nucleophilic addition reactions, which contribute to the biological activities of curcumin [1].

2. Curcumin and disease

Numerous studies in animals and humans over the past several decades have established curcumin outstanding safety and effectiveness against a wide range of diseases where chronic inflammation causes severe pathological conditions, such as cancer, neurological diseases, liver diseases, autoimmune diseases, etc. [2]. For any molecule to be developed as a drug, it should have suitable absorption, distribution, metabolism, and excretion (ADME) properties, which help it to reach therapeutic concentrations at the tissue site after ingestion to exert its effects. But poor water solubility of curcumin, resulting in unsuitable ADME characteristic, which results in low intestinal permeability and adsorption, has become the stumbling block in developing curcumin as a drug. Therefore, efforts to make curcumin bioavailable when delivered through oral route were started. It was realised that for this, curcumin has to be shielded from oxidation and metabolism, and its ability to target diseased tissues should be enhanced. Various natural molecules like piperine, an alkaloid present in *Piper nigrum* Linn., which has been shown to enhance the bioavailability of diverse drugs by inactivating various enzymes on the gut or turmeric oils from *Curcuma longa* rhizome, which has been hypothesised to improve the bioavailability of curcumin, were used. First-generation formulations with enhanced absorption of curcumin were obtained but clinical trials using them did not yield satisfactory results. Then, second-generation formulations using emulsifiers, such as carbohydrate complexes, phospholipid complexes, polysorbates, and water-dispersible nanopreparations, were prepared and tested. These approaches increased curcuminoid levels in the plasma, but most of the curcumin got converted into inactive metabolites like glucuronides and sulphates, limiting clinical efficacy due to their poor tissue penetration and rapid excretion. Therefore, attempts to make third-generation curcumin formulations using the natural curcuminoids and convert them into nanoform without using artificial emulsifiers were made, which improved the bioavailability, membrane permeability, and cellular uptake of curcumin. Therefore using nanoformulations made out of natural curcumin, efforts are being made to find out how they can improve therapeutic efficacy of curcumin and be used in different disease conditions [3].

When curcumin was made into nanoform, its physicochemical characteristics changed, which contributed to its enhanced bioavailability and potency as a therapeutic molecule as compared to conventional curcumin.

Curcumin in the nanoform with greater surface area will have the propensity to bind with proteins, lipids, and polysaccharides avidly as soon as it will be delivered orally and it will resist degradation and will circulate in the blood for longer period of time. It has been shown that under such condition, the metabolism of curcumin in the liver will also be very different.

Analysis by using molecular biology tools has revealed that a large number of cell-signalling molecules have to be dysregulated for manifestation of malignancy. curcumin in the nanoform has been shown to interact with a large number of such cell-signalling molecules, which help tumours to survive and inactivate them. Therefore, circulation of curcumin for a longer period of time would be beneficial as it would prevent the survival and proliferation of the tumours in the body.

3. Curcumin and diet

It has been realised that gut microbiota has an important role in human health and diseases. Therefore, it has emerged as an area of current interest. It is a complex mixture of different organisms, which develop in the gut to fulfil essential physiological functions like providing protection against various infections through maturation of the immune system. It regulates nutritional absorption and metabolism and helps in the production of soluble B vitamins, biotin, folate, etc., which are needed for proper metabolism of the body. Microbiota composition of an individual can change due to ageing and dietary habits. Consumption of unbalanced diets can cause change in gut microbiota composition, which would cause permeability changes and inflammation. Therefore, intake of correct balance of carbohydrates, fats, fibres, etc., in the food is essential for keeping healthy gut, which makes healthy body. There are about 50 bacterial phyla dominated by Bacteroidetes and Firmicutes, and fungi, viruses, and a few other species. The genes of these species when taken together are about 150 times larger than that of the human genome. The most representative species of gut microbiota are *Clostridium*, *Eubacterium*, and *Ruminococcus*, belonging to Firmicutes phyla. It is crucial in determining the abundance of different gut microbial populations [4].

Consumption of curcumin in the diet in the form of turmeric containing only 3–5% curcumin can affect the composition and metabolism of gut microbiome. Using adult healthy volunteers and making them consume moderate quantities of dried *Curcuma longa* extract for 4 weeks, it was observed that urinary fatty acid metabolism changed, indicating a change in the regulation of inflammatory pathways.

It was observed that oral consumption of curcumin alters the ratio between beneficial and harmful bacteria in the gut microbiota community and enhances the function of intestinal barriers like the one containing alkaline phosphatase involved in detoxification of bacterial lipopolysaccharide and mucosa, which inhibits the entry of pathogens into the body.

The interaction between curcumin and gut microbiota is bidirectional, which generates many active metabolites, which are different from what only native curcumin can produce. The net outcome of curcumin entry into the gut therefore will depend on these bioactive metabolites produced by gut microbiota's interaction with curcumin [5].

When trace quantity of curcumin can bring about perceptible changes in the composition and metabolism of gut microbiota, what changes larger quantity of nanoformulation of curcumin with better bioavailability and ability to persist in the tissue when introduced orally into the gut can do has to be considered.

At this stage, a study analysing over 1500 tumour samples from seven cancer types from humans was published. It detected specific bacterial communities within each tumour, which highlighted the presence of a distinct intratumoural microbiome for each tumour, which were resistant to chemotherapy, radiotherapy, and immunotherapy [6]. Therefore, it became clear that killing the cancer cells within this tumour microbiome will depend upon the ability of the therapeutic agent to disrupt the immunosuppressive environment maintained by the cancer cells inside the tumour microbiome. Therefore, efforts should continue to find out conditions under which curcumin molecule along with the metabolites generated by the gut microbiome can penetrate the tumour microbiome and alter the immunosuppressive environment, which protects the cancer cells.

Author details

Santosh K. Kar
KIIT Technology Business Incubator, Kalinga Institute of Industrial Technology, Bhubaneswar, Odisha, India

*Address all correspondence to: santoshkar1946@gmail.com

References

[1] Jamil SNH et al. Curcumin and its derivatives as potential antimalarial and anti-inflammatory agents: A review on structure-activity relationship and mechanism of action. Pharmaceuticals (Basel). 2023;**16**(4):609. DOI: 10.3390/ph16040609

[2] Aggarwal BB, Harikumar KB. Potential therapeutic effects of curcumin, the anti-inflammatory agent, against neurodegenerative, cardiovascular, pulmonary, metabolic, autoimmune and neoplastic diseases. The International Journal of Biochemistry & Cell Biology. 2009;**41**(1):40-59. DOI: 10.1016/j.biocel.2008.06.010

[3] Hegde M et al. Curcumin formulations for better bioavailability: What we learned from clinical trials thus far? ACS Omega. 2023;**8**(12):10713-10746. DOI: 10.1021/acsomega.2c07326

[4] Hills RD Jr et al. Gut microbiome: Profound implications for diet and disease. Nutrients. 2019;**11**(7):1613. DOI: 10.3390/nu11071613

[5] Balaji S et al. Impact of curcumin on gut microbiome. World Journal of Experimental Medicine. 2025;**15**(1):100275. DOI: 10.5493/wjem.v15.i1.100275

[6] Battaglia TW et al. A pan-cancer analysis of the microbiome in metastatic cancer. Cell. 2024;**187**(9):2324-2335.e19. DOI: 10.1016/j.cell.2024.03.021

Chapter 2

Chemical and Physical Properties, Pharmacokinetics, and Pharmacodynamics of Curcumin Derivatives

Galih Satrio Putra, Muhammad Ainur Hasan,
Melanny Ika Sulistyowaty, Farida Anwari and Dini Kesuma

Abstract

Curcumin derivatives (Curcuminoids) are a highly intriguing class of phytochemical compounds, widely discussed due to their presence as active ingredients in various pharmaceutical formulations and food supplements. There are three main compounds in curcuminoids: curcumin, desmethoxycurcumin, and bisdemethoxycurcumin. These compounds exhibit distinct chemical structures, which significantly influence their chemical and physical properties, pharmacokinetic profiles, and pharmacodynamic characteristics. From a pharmacokinetic perspective, curcuminoid-based formulations present unique challenges due to their poor water solubility and low permeability in the gastrointestinal tract (GIT). In terms of pharmacodynamics, curcuminoids interact with multiple receptor targets and enzymes, contributing to a wide range of pharmacological effects, including anti-inflammatory, antioxidant, and anticancer activities, among others. Therefore, this book explores in depth the chemical and physical properties of curcumin derivatives and their impact on pharmacokinetic and pharmacodynamic profiles.

Keywords: curcuminoid, curcumin, desmethoxycurcumin, bisdemethoxycurcumin, chemical–physical properties, pharmacokinetics, pharmacodynamics

1. Introduction

Curcuminoids belong to a class of secondary metabolites/phytochemical compounds, similar to other phytochemical groups such as flavonoids, alkaloids, and terpenoids. The biosynthetic pathway of curcuminoid compounds in Curcuma sp. [1, 2] originates from the primary metabolite L-phenylalanine (1), which undergoes deamination to form cinnamic acid (2). Cinnamic acid (2) serves as the starting material for the synthesis of coumaric acid (3), caffeic acid (4), and ferulic acid (5). Ferulic acid is synthesized from coumaric acid through the intermediate product, caffeic acid

(4). Both coumaric acid (3) and ferulic acid (5) are the main precursors in the formation of the curcuminoid framework. Coumaric acid (3) is converted by the enzyme 4CL (4-coumarate-CoA ligase) into the more reactive compound coumaroyl-CoA (6). Similarly, ferulic acid (5) is converted by the same enzyme into feruloyl-CoA (7), which is also a more reactive compound. Coumaroyl-CoA (6) and feruloyl-CoA (7) then react with the acid group from malonyl-CoA to form coumaroyl-diketide-CoA (9) and feruloyl-diketide-CoA (10) with the assistance of the enzyme DSC (diketide-CoA synthase). Coumaroyl-diketide-CoA (9) reacts with ferulic acid (5) to form demethoxycurcumin (10) with the help of the CURs (curcumin synthases) enzyme. Similarly, feruloyl-diketide-CoA (10) reacts with coumaric acid (3) under the action of CURs to produce demethoxycurcumin (10). If coumaroyl-diketide-CoA (9) reacts with coumaric acid (3), it forms bisdemethoxycurcumin (11), while feruloyl-diketide-CoA (10) reacts with ferulic acid (5) results in the formation of curcumin. Thus, the biosynthetic pathway of curcuminoids (curcumin, demethoxycurcumin, and bisdemethoxycurcumin) is illustrated in **Figure 1**.

Curcuminoids are phytochemical compounds widely found in Curcuma species, such as *Curcuma longa* (Turmeric), *Curcuma xanthorrhiza* (Javanese Ginger), *Curcuma heyneana* (Javanese Giring Ginger), *Curcuma zedoaria* (White Turmeric), etc. [3]. There are three main compounds classified as curcuminoids: curcumin, demethoxycurcumin, and bisdemethoxycurcumin, whose chemical structures are presented in **Figure 2**.

The curcuminoid content in Curcuma species can serve as both an identity marker and a pharmacological activity marker. For example, extraction using 90% ethanol as a solvent from *Curcuma longa* (Turmeric) and *Curcuma heyneana* (Javanese Giring Ginger) contains three curcuminoids: curcumin, demethoxycurcumin, and

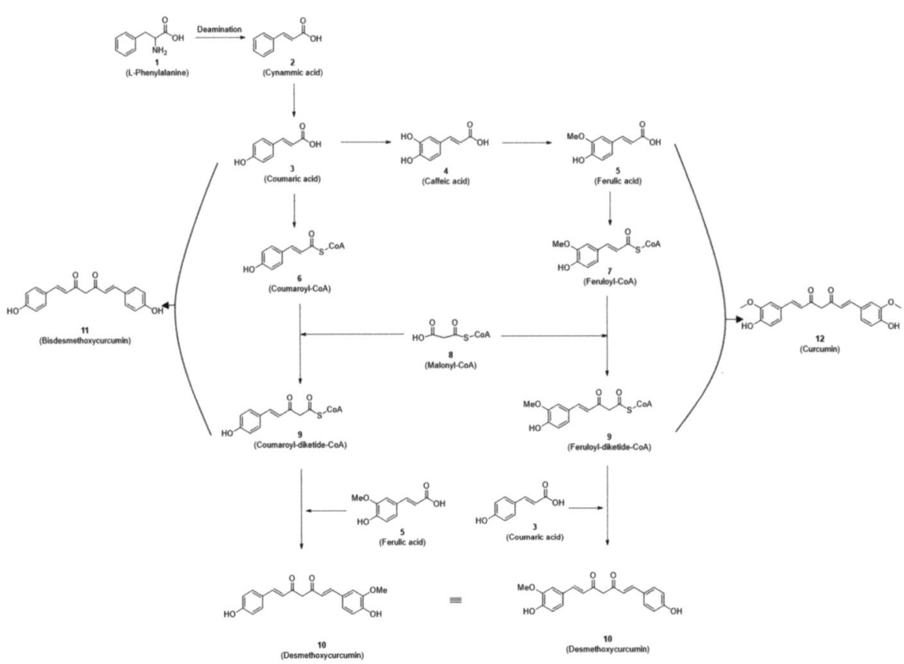

Figure 1.
Biosynthesis of curcuminoid (curcumin, demethoxycurcumin, and bisdemethoxycurcumin) in Curcuma sp.

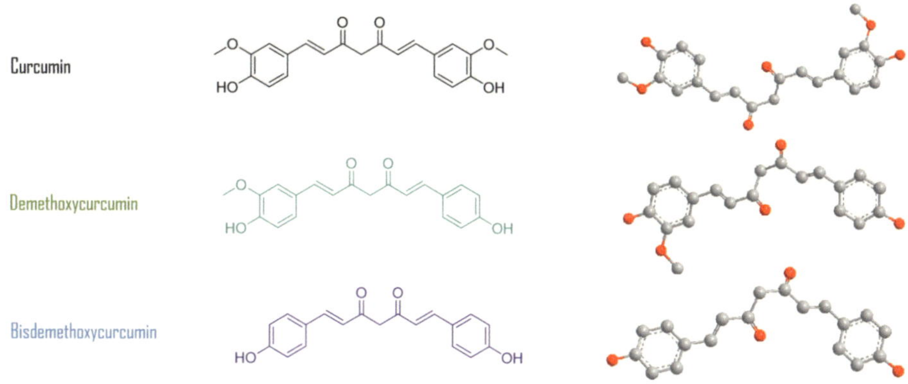

Figure 2.
2D and 3D chemical structure of curcuminoid (curcumin, demethoxycurcumin, and bisdemethoxycurcumin).

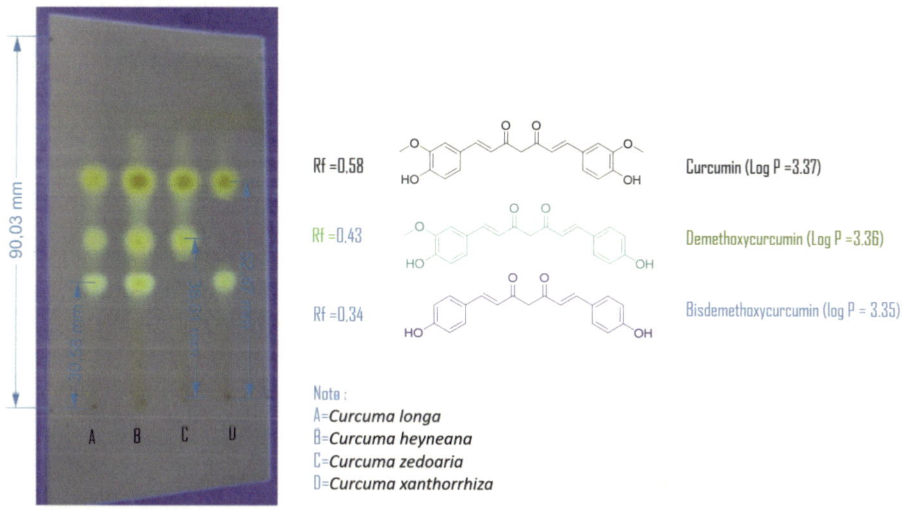

Figure 3.
TLC Profile of Curcuminoid under UV light at 366 nm, using a stationary phase of Silica Gel 60 GF 256 and a mobile phase of chloroform: ethanol: glacial acetic acid (94:5:1).

bisdemethoxycurcumin. However, extraction with 90% ethanol from *Curcuma xanthorrhiza* (Javanese Ginger) contains only two curcuminoids, there are curcumin and demethoxycurcumin. Similarly, *Curcuma zedoaria* (White Turmeric) also contains only two curcuminoids: curcumin and desmethoxycurcumin. These differences can be observed through Thin Layer Chromatography (TLC) under UV light at 366 nm, using a stationary phase of Silica Gel 60 GF 256 and a mobile phase of chloroform: ethanol: glacial acetic acid (94:5:1), as illustrated in **Figure 3** [4].

2. Chemical and physical properties of curcuminoids

The major phytochemicals of curcuminoids are curcumin, demethoxycurcumin, and bisdemethoxycurcumin. The distinguishing factor among them is the presence or absence of methoxy groups. Methoxy groups are auxochromes that are nonpolar and act as electron-donating groups, which can activate the benzene ring. The presence of methoxy groups significantly influences the chemical and physical properties of curcuminoids, including lipophilicity, solubility, melting point, antioxidant activity, and acidity [5–7].

2.1 Lipophilicity of curcuminoids (Log P)

The loss of one or two methoxy groups in curcumin results in distinct chemical and physical properties, which in turn lead to different pharmacokinetic and pharmacodynamic profiles. A simple example is the separation of curcumin (Log P = 3.369), demethoxycurcumin (Log P = 3.361), and bisdemethoxycurcumin (Log P = 3.353) using Thin Layer Chromatography (TLC) with a polar stationary phase, Silica Gel 60 GF 256, and a nonpolar mobile phase consisting of chloroform: ethanol: acetic glacial (94:5:1) due to their significantly different polarities [4, 8].

Methoxy groups are nonpolar, so the loss of methoxy groups increases polarity, leading to a lower Log P and a higher Log S compared to curcumin. As a result, the polarity ranking is bisdemethoxycurcumin > demethoxycurcumin > curcumin, whereas their lipophilicity follows the opposite trend: curcumin > demethoxycurcumin > bisdemethoxycurcumin [9].

This phenomenon causes bisdemethoxycurcumin to have the smallest Rf value (0.34) among the three, as its higher polarity allows stronger interactions with the stationary phase (silica gel), which contains silanol groups, as shown in **Figure 4**. In contrast, curcumin is more eluted by the nonpolar mobile phase, giving it the highest Rf value (0.58). This occurs because curcumin dissolves better in the nonpolar mobile phase due to the presence of two methoxy groups. Additionally, these two methoxy groups create steric hindrance between the silanol groups of the silica gel and the phenolic alcohol or beta-diketone groups in curcumin, weakening hydrogen bond interactions compared to bisdemethoxycurcumin (**Figure 4**).

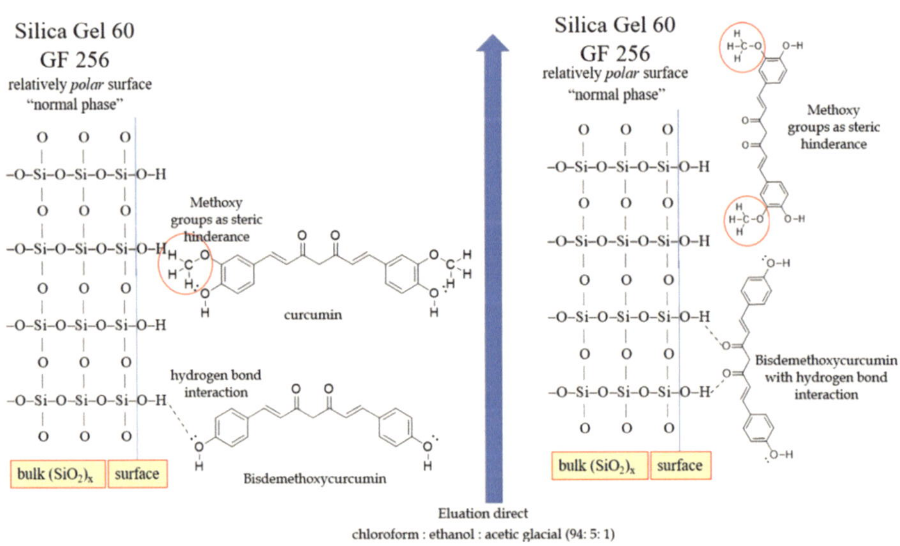

Figure 4.
Chemical bond interaction between curcuminoids with the stationary phase of Silica Gel 60 GF 256 and a mobile phase of chloroform: ethanol: glacial acetic acid (94:5:1).

2.2 Solubility of curcuminoids (Log S)

The solubility of curcuminoids in water falls under the classification of practically insoluble (<0.1 mg/mL). However, in terms of their relative solubility in water, bisdemethoxycurcumin (0.015 mg/mL) > demethoxycurcumin (6.56×10^{-3} mg/mL) > curcumin (3.5×10^{-3} mg/mL) [8]. The loss of two nonpolar (-OMe) groups allows bisdemethoxycurcumin to interact more easily with water molecules through hydrogen bonding compared to curcumin. The presence of nonpolar methoxy groups hinders water molecules from forming hydrogen bonds with the phenolic groups of curcumin due to steric hindrance, resulting in a solubility of approximately 3.5×10^{-3} mg/mL in water for curcumin, whereas bisdemethoxycurcumin has a solubility of about 0.015 mg/mL. This phenomenon is illustrated in **Figure 5**.

The presence or absence of methoxy groups also affects the Log S values of curcuminoids. Log S represents the logarithm of a compound's partition coefficient in water/octanol, indicating its solubility behavior: the higher the Log S (+) value, the more soluble the compound is in polar solvents (water) [10–12]. Conversely, a lower Log S (−) value indicates reduced solubility in polar solvents (water). The Log S values of bisdemethoxycurcumin (Log S = −4.23) > demethoxycurcumin (Log S = −4.34) > curcumin (Log S = −4.45), as bisdemethoxycurcumin can interact more readily with water molecules through hydrogen bonding compared to curcumin [11, 12].

Curcuminoids, which fall under the category of practically insoluble in water, require the use of solvents with higher solubility for the extraction process from Curcuma species. Researchers commonly use ethanol, acetone, or DMSO as extraction solvents due to their superior solubility properties. Curcuminoids exhibit solubility in 96% ethanol and acetone at approximately 33–100 mg/mL and are highly soluble in DMSO at concentrations >1000 mg/mL. This is because DMSO is a polar aprotic solvent known for its ability to effectively dissolve many organic compounds [13].

2.3 Melting point of curcuminoids

Curcumin has a melting point of 183°C, whereas bisdemethoxycurcumin has a melting point of 233°C [14–16]. The higher melting point of bisdemethoxycurcumin compared to curcumin is due to the absence of two methoxy groups, which facilitates the formation of stronger intramolecular hydrogen bonds. As a result, a higher amount of thermal energy is required to break these bonds and transition from the solid to the liquid phase. In contrast, curcumin has difficulty forming intramolecular

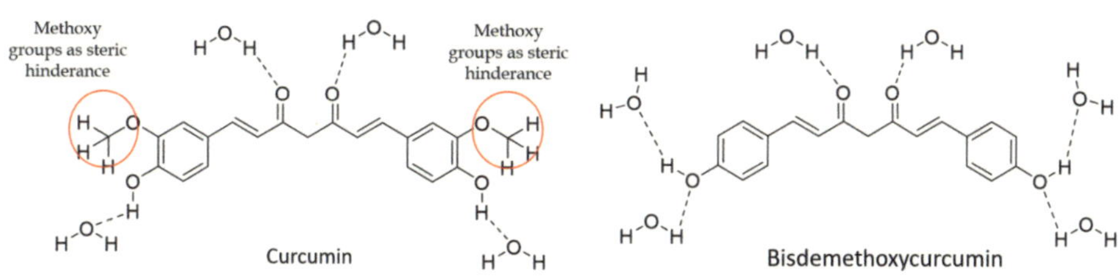

Figure 5.
Hydrogen bond interaction between curcuminoid and water.

hydrogen bonds due to the presence of two methoxy groups, which introduce steric hindrance, as illustrated in **Figure 6**. When ranked by melting point values, the order is: Bisdemethoxycurcumin > Demethoxycurcumin > Curcumin.

2.4 Antioxidant activity of curcuminoids

The antioxidant mechanism to counteract reactive oxygen species (ROS) consists of primary and secondary antioxidants [3, 17–18]. Primary antioxidants function to stop the formation of free radicals or capture free radicals before they cause further damage. The main mechanism of primary antioxidants is to scavenge free radicals and stabilize them by donating electrons without becoming reactive free radicals themselves or inhibiting the free radical chain reaction by converting free radicals into a less reactive form.

Secondary antioxidants work by supporting the function of primary antioxidants or deactivating free radical products that have already formed. Secondary antioxidants do not directly scavenge free radicals but inhibit oxidative reactions through various mechanisms. The main mechanisms of secondary antioxidants include chelating heavy metal transitions such as Cu^{2+}, Pb^{2+}, and Ni^{2+}, or regenerating primary antioxidants and breaking down ROS [3, 17–19].

Curcuminoid compounds exhibit both primary and secondary antioxidant activities. The primary antioxidant activity of curcuminoids occurs through free radical scavenging and stabilization via the resonance system present in their structure. Curcumin has the best resonance stability compared to bisdemethoxycurcumin and demethoxycurcumin because it possesses two methoxy groups, which act as Electron-Donating Groups (EDGs) that donate electrons to the conjugated system or aromatic ring [5–7]. The presence of two methoxy groups activates the aromatic ring, making it more ∂^- (partially negative), which aligns with the resonance system, thereby facilitating the release of hydrogen atoms from its two phenolic groups to neutralize ROS, as illustrated in **Figure 7**.

Additionally, the presence of two methoxy groups induces a latent polarity system (**Figure 8**) that aligns with the resonance system, allowing for more effective neutralization of ROS compared to bisdemethoxycurcumin and demethoxycurcumin [20, 21].

For this reason, curcumin exhibits a higher potential as an antioxidant compared to bisdemethoxycurcumin and demethoxycurcumin. When ranked by antioxidant potential, the order is as follows: Curcumin > Demethoxycurcumin > Bisdemethoxycurcumin.

Based on in vitro antioxidant activity assays using the DPPH method, it has been reported that the IC_{50} values are 4.7 μM for curcumin, 5.2 μM for

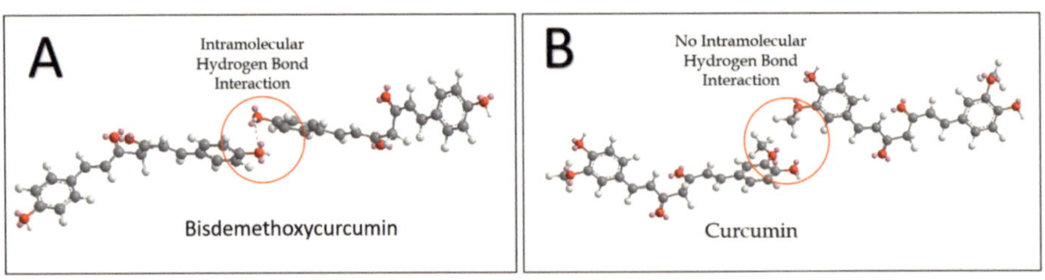

Figure 6.
Intramolecular hydrogen bond interaction: A. Bisdemethoxycurcumin; B. Curcumin.

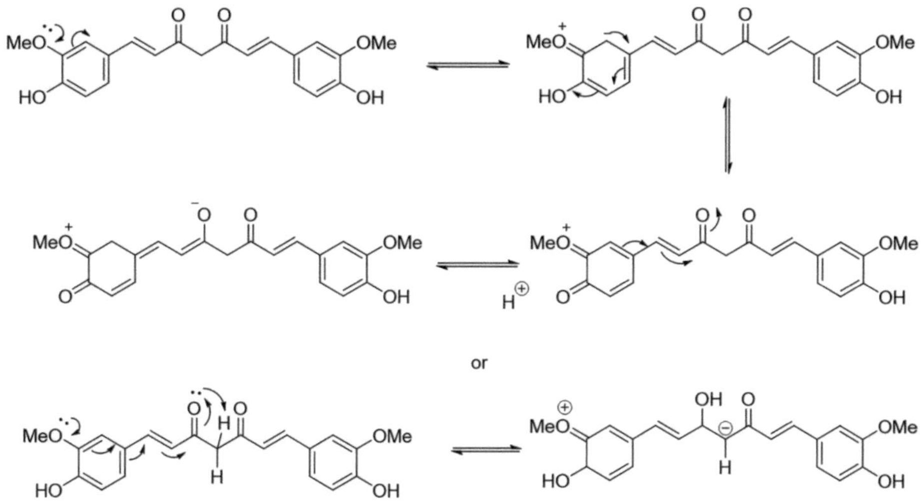

Figure 7.
Resonance system in the chemical structure of curcuminoid.

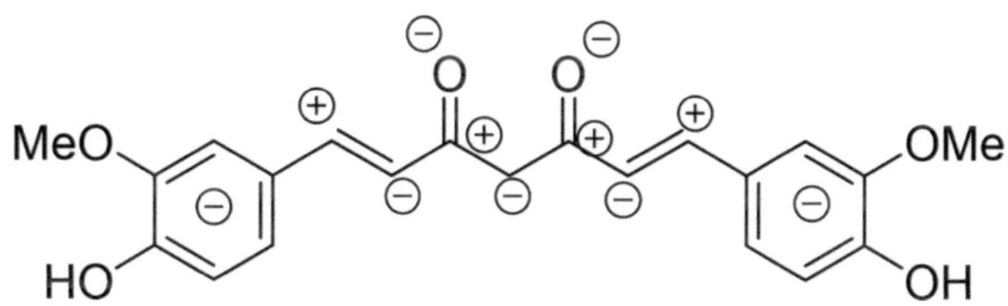

Figure 8.
Latent polarity in the curcuminoid system.

demethoxycurcumin, and 7.0 μM for bisdemethoxycurcumin [3, 17–19]. The process of free radical stabilization by curcumin is illustrated in **Figure 9**.

The secondary antioxidant activity of curcuminoids has been widely reported for their ability to chelate several heavy metal transition ions, such as Hg^{2+}, Pb^{2+}, Cu^{2+}, Ni^{2+}, etc. [19]. The presence of methoxy groups in curcumin induces a repulsion effect, creating space for chelating heavy metal transition ions, making the chelation process more stable compared to bisdemethoxycurcumin and demethoxycurcumin, as illustrated in **Figure 10**.

2.5 Acidity of curcuminoid (pKa)

The presence or absence of methoxy groups in curcuminoids leads to differences in pKa values. A lower pKa value indicates that a compound is more prone to protonation or the release of H+, meaning it exhibits stronger acidity [5–7]. The influence of methoxy groups on acidity can be observed in **Table 1**. Methoxy groups, classified as Electron Donating Groups (EDG), activate the aromatic ring, making the hydrogen atom on the phenolic group more easily dissociable [22]. This is evident in curcumin, where the presence of methoxy groups results in a phenolic hydrogen pKa value of 9.4, whereas in the absence of methoxy groups, the pKa value

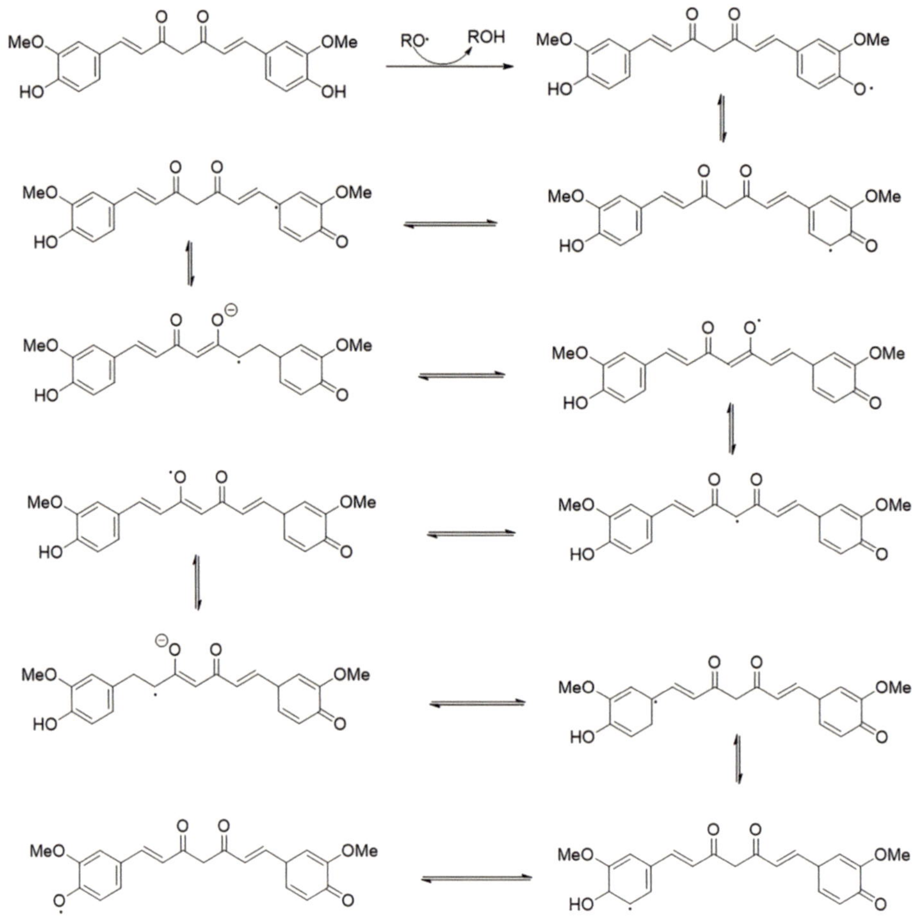

Figure 9.
Mechanism of Radical Oxygen Species (ROS) neutralization in the chemical structure of curcumin.

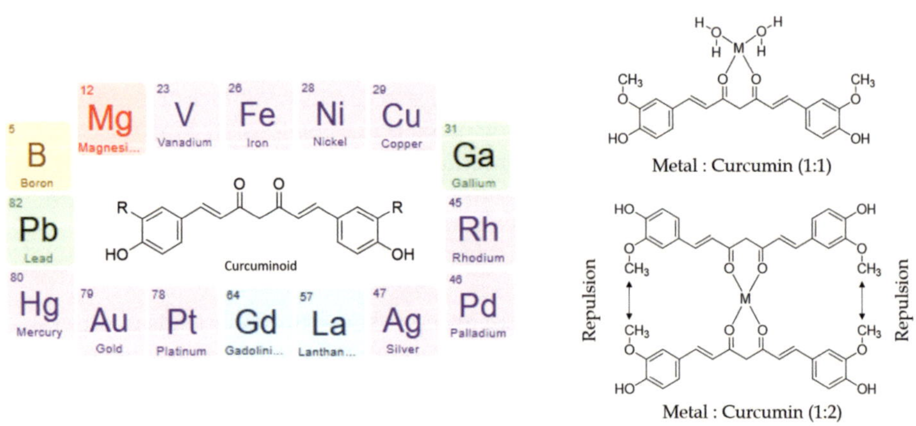

Figure 10.
Chelation process of curcumin with various metal elements.

Compounds	H atoms position	pKa
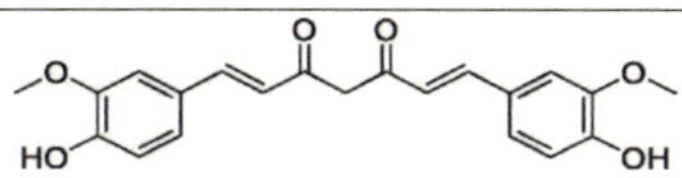 Curcumin	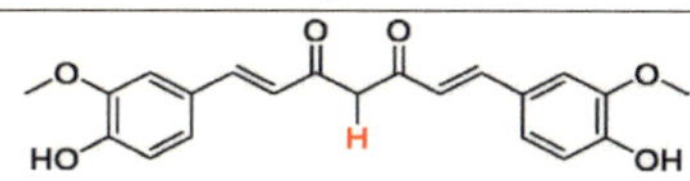	8.1
	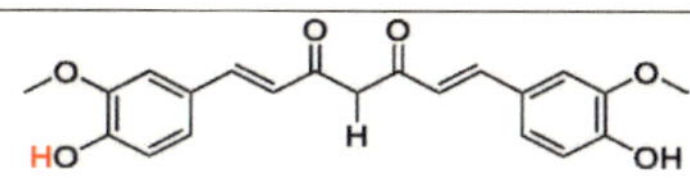	9.4
	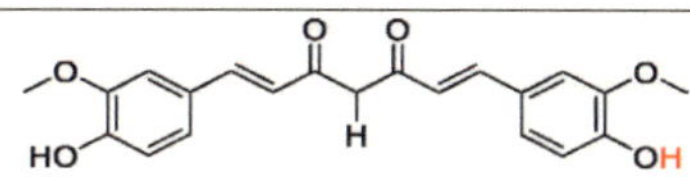	9.4
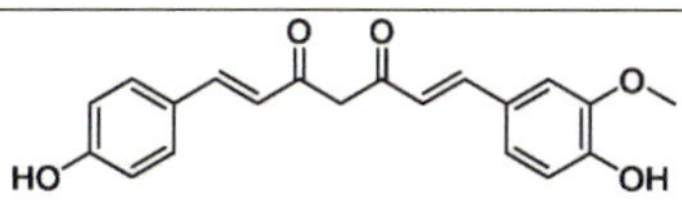 Demethoxycurcumin	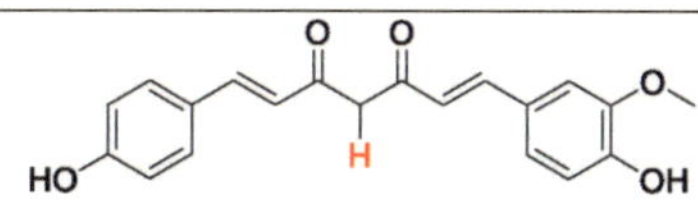	8.2
	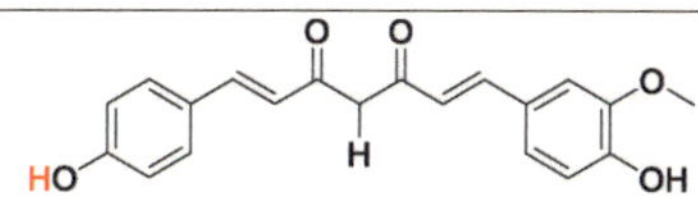	9.6
	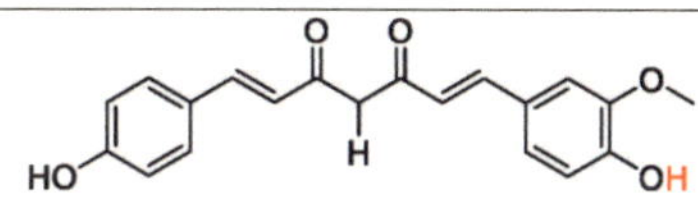	9.4
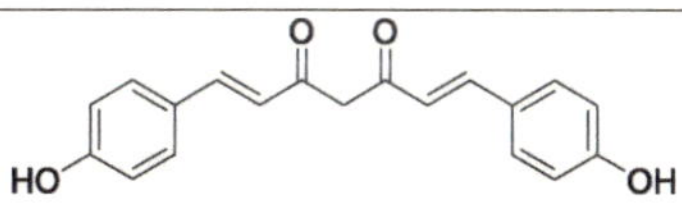 Bisdemethoxycurcumin	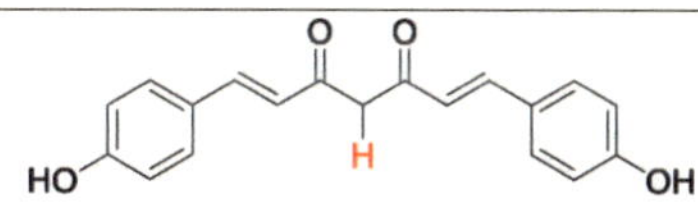	8.3
	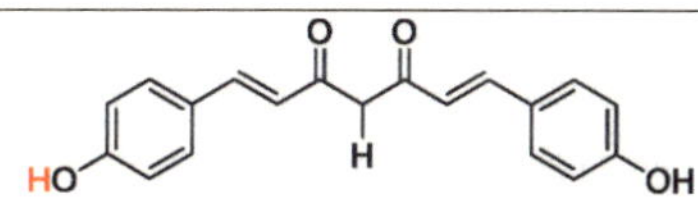	9.6
	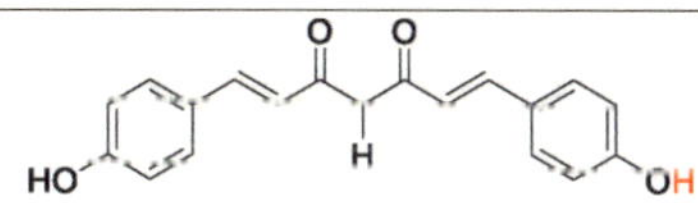	9.6

Table 1.
pKa values of acidic hydrogen atoms.

of the phenolic hydrogen remains 9.4 [22]. The methoxy groups not only activate the benzene ring but also contribute to resonance effects within the diketone system, facilitating the dissociation of the α-hydrogen. This is reflected in the pKa values of curcumin (8.1), demethoxycurcumin (8.2), and bisdemethoxycurcumin (8.3). The overall resonance effects influenced by methoxy groups are illustrated in **Figure 7**.

3. Pharmacokinetics of curcuminoids

The differences in the chemical and physical properties of curcumin, demethoxycurcumin, and bisdemethoxycurcumin, resulting from variations in their chemical structures, also impact their pharmacokinetic aspects, including absorption, distribution, metabolism, and excretion. These differences are discussed in detail one by one.

3.1 Absorption of curcuminoids

To determine how well curcuminoids are absorbed through the gastrointestinal tract (GIT), it is necessary to compare their water solubility and permeability data [10, 23]. Both of these factors play a crucial role in determining the Biopharmaceutical Classification System (BCS) category to which they belong. The water solubility and permeability data of curcuminoids are presented in **Table 2**.

Curcumin has poor water solubility (low solubility) and falls into the category of practically insoluble, with a solubility of <0.1 mg/mL. Its permeability is 4.87×10^{-6} cm/s, which is classified as low permeability since it is $<9.0 \times 10^{-6}$ cm/s [8, 24, 25]. Curcumin belongs to BCS Class IV because it has both low solubility and low permeability (**Figure 11**) [10]. BCS Class IV compounds exhibit very poor bioavailability when absorbed through the gastrointestinal tract (GIT). Several in vivo studies have shown that oral administration of a single 2 g dose of curcumin in Mus musculus resulted in plasma concentrations of less than 5 μg/mL, indicating poor absorption in the GIT [26].

The removal of one methoxy group from curcumin results in demethoxycurcumin. Since the methoxy group is nonpolar, its absence slightly increases water solubility to 6.56×10^{-3} mg/mL. However, the solubility of demethoxycurcumin is still classified as low solubility and remains in the practically insoluble category (<0.1 mg/mL) [10, 23]. The loss of one methoxy group significantly affects the permeability of demethoxycurcumin, which has a permeability value of 12.53×10^{-6} cm/s, classifying it as high permeability since it is $>9.0 \times 10^{-6}$ cm/s [8, 24, 25]. Demethoxycurcumin falls into BCS Class II due to its low solubility and high permeability (**Figure 11**). BCS Class II compounds exhibit slightly higher bioavailability compared to curcumin.

The removal of two methoxy groups from curcumin results in bisdemethoxycurcumin. Since methoxy groups are nonpolar, their absence slightly increases water solubility to 0.015 mg/mL. However, bisdemethoxycurcumin still falls into the low

Compounds	Water solubility (mg/ml)	Coca2 permeability (cm/s)	BCS class
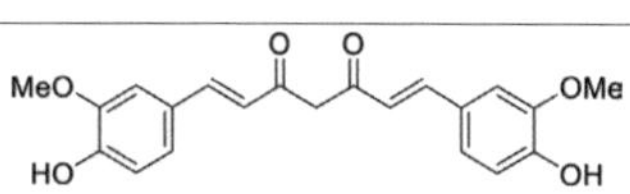 Curcumin	3.5×10^{-3} Practically insoluble	4.87×10^{-6} Low permeability	IV
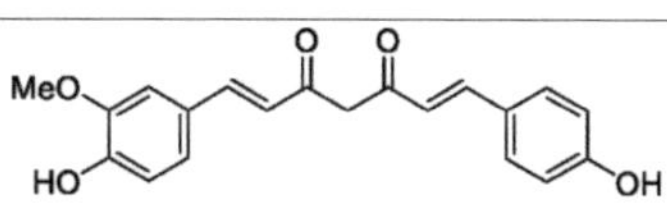 Demethoxycurcumin	6.56×10^{-3} Practically insoluble	12.53×10^{-6} High permeability	II
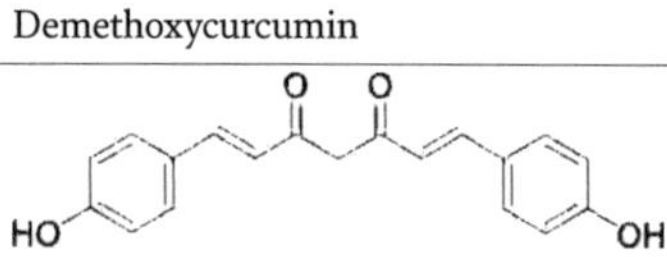 Bisdemethoxycurcumin	0.015 Practically insoluble	12.56×10^{-6} High permeability	II

Table 2.
Data on water solubility, permeability, and BCS of curcuminoids.

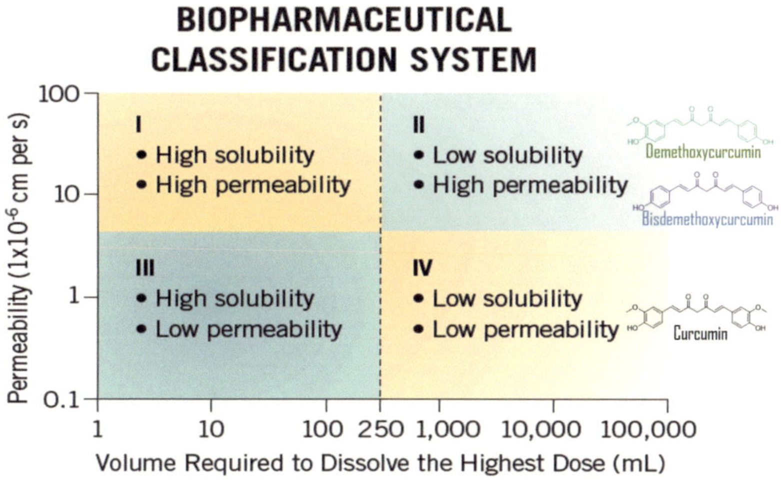

Figure 11.
Biopharmaceuticals classification system quadrant of curcuminoids.

solubility category and remains classified as practically insoluble (<0.1 mg/mL) [10, 23]. The loss of two methoxy groups significantly influences the permeability of bisdemethoxycurcumin, which has a permeability value of 12.56 × 10^{-6} cm/s, classifying it as high permeability (>9.0 × 10^{-6} cm/s) [8, 24, 25]. Bisdemethoxycurcumin belongs to BCS Class II due to its low solubility and high permeability (**Figure 11**). Among curcumin and its derivatives, bisdemethoxycurcumin has the highest bioavailability. Therefore, in terms of bioavailability, the ranking from highest to lowest is as follows: Bisdemethoxycurcumin > Demethoxycurcumin > Curcumin.

3.2 Distribution of curcuminoids

Curcuminoids are natural compounds classified as weak acids [13]. Weakly acidic compounds tend to bind to albumin proteins, whereas weakly basic compounds are more likely to interact with P-glycoprotein [27–29]. Curcumin contains methoxy groups that act as Electron Donating Groups (EDG), activating the benzene ring and making the alpha hydrogen in the diketone system more prone to releasing H+, thereby generating a negative charge on the curcumin molecule. This negative charge facilitates its binding to albumin proteins (**Figure 12**).

Several studies have reported that curcumin binds to plasma albumin proteins at a rate of more than 95% [30–32]. When curcumin interacts with albumin, it has a longer half-life, takes more time to be metabolized, and requires a longer duration for excretion from the body [27]. However, it is also important to consider its interactions with other drugs that bind to albumin, as curcumin may displace them, leading to an increase in free drug concentration in the blood [27–29]. As of now, moderate interactions between curcumin and 132 drugs have been documented on the website www.drugs.com, which is widely used by clinicians to identify drug–drug interactions when medications are administered concurrently [33, 34]. Based on the binding affinity of curcuminoids to plasma albumin proteins, the order is as follows: curcumin > demethoxycurcumin > bisdemethoxycurcumin.

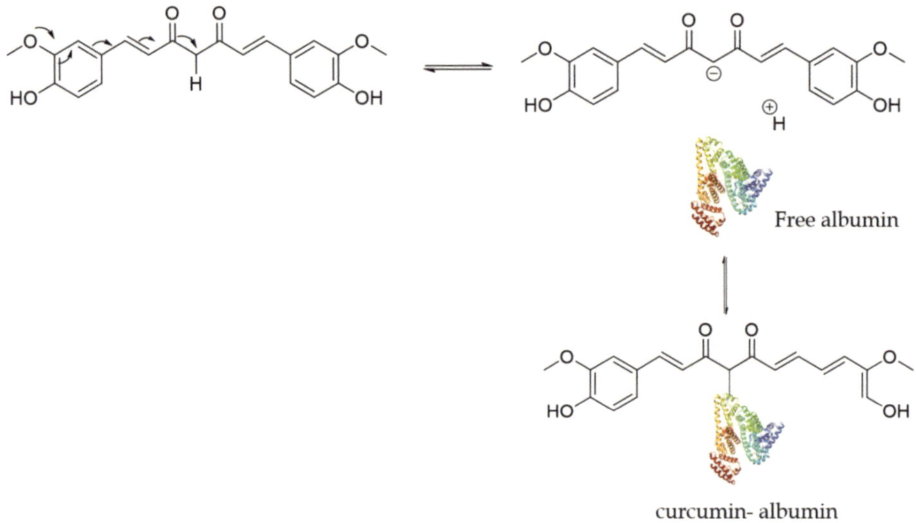

Figure 12.
Curcumin-albumin chemical bonding interaction.

3.3 Metabolism of curcuminoids

The primary purpose of curcuminoid metabolism in the liver is to convert lipophilic curcuminoids into hydrophilic compounds, allowing them to be excreted through the kidneys [27]. The metabolism of curcuminoids transforms active compounds into inactive metabolites. There are two phases in curcuminoid metabolism: phase 1 and phase 2 [27–29]. Phase 1 begins with the metabolism of curcuminoids into slightly more polar compounds [27]. Several studies have reported that curcuminoids undergo demethylation and reduction reactions during phase 1 metabolism [3, 18, 35].

Curcumin undergoes phase 1 metabolism through demethylation and reduction processes. The demethylation process converts curcumin into demethylcurcumin. Since curcumin contains two methoxy groups, further demethylation leads to the formation of bisdemethylcurcumin [3]. During the reduction process, curcumin is converted into tetrahydrocurcumin, followed by hexahydrocurcumin, and then further reduced to hexahydrocurcuminol (**Figure 13**).

In phase 1 metabolism, curcumin is transformed into slightly polar metabolites. As a result, these metabolites are rarely found in urine but are more commonly excreted in feces alongside bile salts [14]. These metabolites participate in the enterohepatic cycle, which plays a role in dissolving gallstones in cases of cholestasis [14].

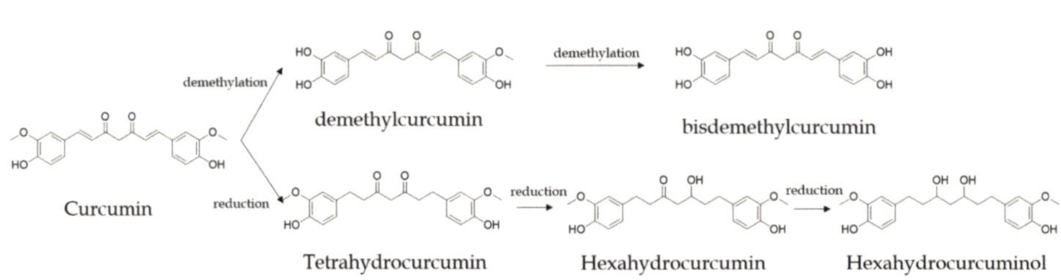

Figure 13.
Phase 1 metabolism of curcumin.

Demethoxycurcumin also undergoes phase 1 metabolism through methylation and reduction processes [3]. However, due to the loss of one methoxy group, the methylation process occurs in only one step, resulting in demethyldemethoxycurcumin. Meanwhile, the reduction process remains the same, producing three major metabolites: tetrahydrodemethoxycurcumin, hexahydrodemethoxycurcumin, and hexahydrodemethoxycurcuminol (**Figure 14**).

During phase 1 metabolism, demethoxycurcumin is converted into slightly polar metabolites. As a result, these metabolites are rarely found in urine but are more commonly excreted in feces along with bile salts. These metabolites participate in the enterohepatic cycle, which plays a role in dissolving gallstones in cases of cholestasis.

Bisdemethoxycurcumin undergoes phase 1 metabolism exclusively through the reduction process without methylation, as it lacks methoxy groups entirely, as shown in **Figure 14**. Bisdemethoxycurcumin is reduced into three major metabolites: tetrahydrobisdemethoxycurcumin, hexahydrobisdemethoxycurcumin, and hexahydrobisdemethoxycurcuminol (**Figure 15**) [3].

During phase 1 metabolism, bisdemethoxycurcumin is converted into slightly polar metabolites. As a result, these metabolites are rarely found in urine but are more commonly excreted in feces along with bile salts. These metabolites participate in the enterohepatic cycle, which plays a role in dissolving gallstones in cases of cholestasis [14].

Phase 2 metabolism of curcuminoids occurs through sulfate conjugation and glucuronic acid conjugation, as illustrated in **Figure 16**. In this phase, curcumin is converted into curcumin sulfate and curcumin glucuronide [3, 18, 35]. The sulfate and glucuronic conjugation processes in curcumin are more challenging due to the presence of two methoxy groups, which create steric hindrance. This steric effect slows down the metabolism compared to bisdemethoxycurcumin, which lacks methoxy groups [5–7].

For demethoxycurcumin, the sulfate and glucuronic conjugation processes produce demethoxycurcumin sulfate and demethoxycurcumin glucuronide. These reactions occur faster than in curcumin because the absence of one methoxy group reduces steric hindrance, facilitating the attachment of sulfate and glucuronic acid groups. In contrast, bisdemethoxycurcumin undergoes sulfate and glucuronic

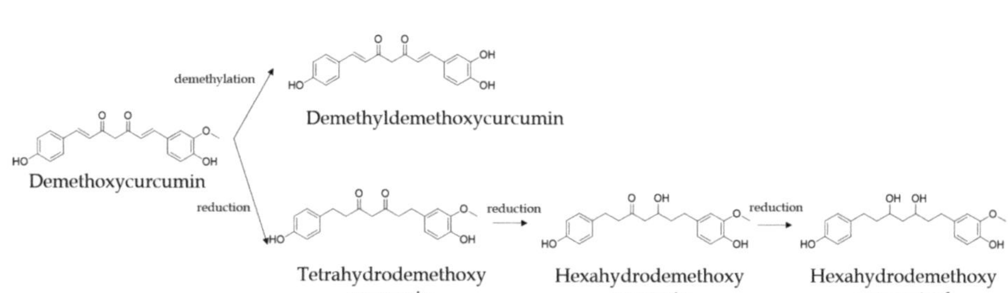

Figure 14.
Phase 1 metabolism of demethoxycurcumin.

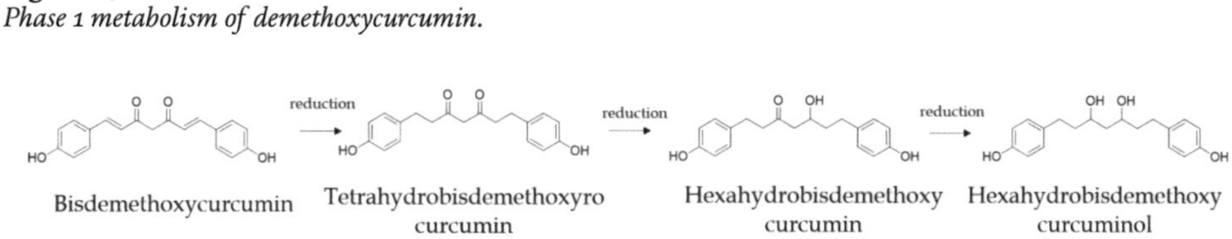

Figure 15.
Phase 1 metabolism of bisdemethoxycurcumin.

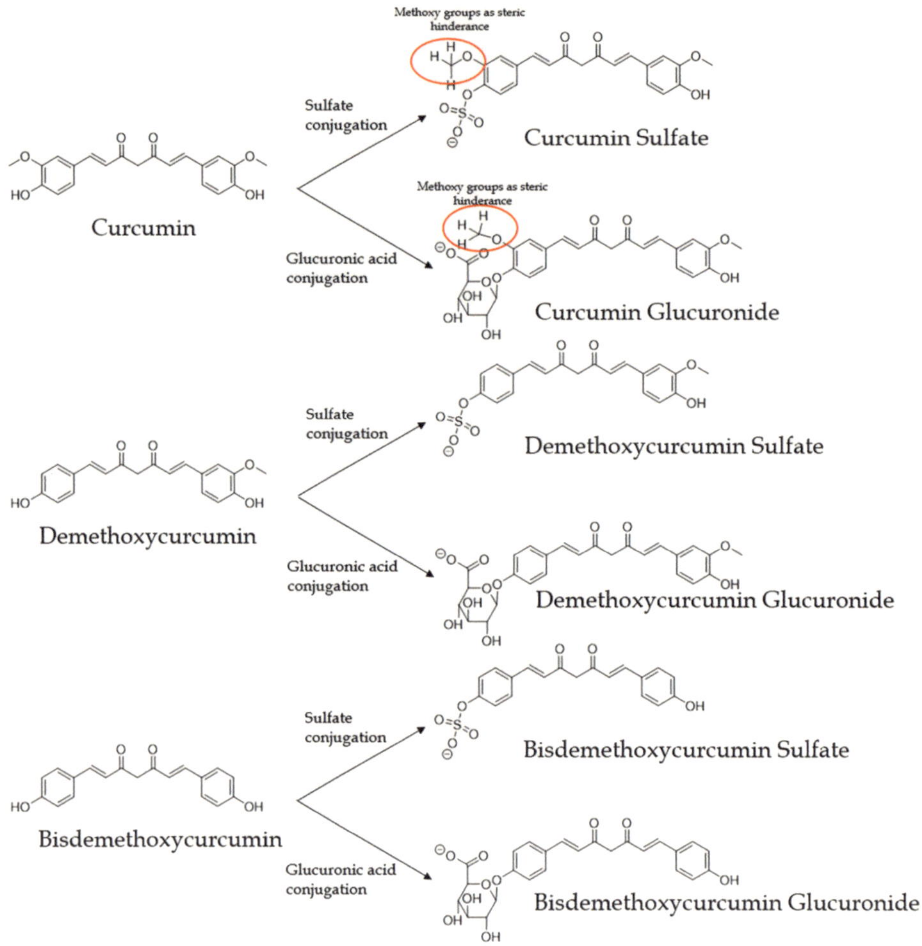

Figure 16.
Phase 2 metabolism of curcuminoids.

conjugation even more rapidly, producing bisdemethoxycurcumin sulfate and bisdemethoxycurcumin glucuronide.

The complete absence of methoxy groups allows easier attachment of sulfate and glucuronic acid, increasing the likelihood of conjugation. Sulfate and glucuronic acid groups are highly polar due to their anionic charges, making them highly water-soluble [5–7]. Consequently, the phase 2 metabolism of curcuminoids produces very polar metabolites that can be easily excreted through the kidneys in urine [14].

The metabolic rate of curcuminoids ranked from the slowest to the fastest, is as follows: Curcumin > Demethoxycurcumin > Bisdemethoxycurcumin. The presence of two methoxy groups in curcumin not only enhances its binding to albumin, prolonging its metabolism but also introduces steric hindrance, delaying sulfate and glucuronic acid conjugation.

3.4 Excretion of curcuminoids

Curcuminoids are eliminated from the body through two organs: the liver and kidneys [27]. The majority of phase 1 curcuminoid metabolites are excreted via the liver

[14, 27]. More than 90% of curcumin is excreted in feces through the enterohepatic cycle, while a smaller portion is excreted in urine [14, 27]. This phenomenon occurs because the presence of two methoxy groups in curcumin facilitates its metabolism via phase 1 through methylation and reduction, producing slightly polar metabolites that are stored in bile salts, secreted into the gastrointestinal tract, and eliminated with feces. The high concentration of curcumin in bile makes it more effective in dissolving gallstones in cholestasis cases compared to demethoxycurcumin and bisdemethoxycurcumin.

A small portion of curcumin undergoes phase 2 metabolism through sulfate conjugation and glucuronic conjugation. However, the presence of two methoxy groups creates significant steric hindrance, which interferes with these processes, resulting in fewer metabolites and consequently lower urinary excretion of curcumin. Some studies report that curcumin has a half-life ($t_1/_2$) of 6.77 ± 0.83 hours [35], while others report a half-life of 7–8 hours [36]. Curcumin's half-life falls within the intermediate half-life category (4–12 hours), with a recommended administration of 1–2 times per day.

Compared to curcumin, demethoxycurcumin, and bisdemethoxycurcumin have shorter half-lives due to the absence of methoxy groups, which accelerate phase 1 and phase 2 metabolism. Bisdemethoxycurcumin is more easily excreted in urine by the kidneys. The lack of methoxy groups allows bisdemethoxycurcumin to undergo phase 2 metabolism more rapidly through sulfate conjugation and glucuronic conjugation, producing highly polar metabolites that are easily dissolved in urine. This phenomenon results in bisdemethoxycurcumin having a shorter excretion half-life ($t_1/_2$) compared to demethoxycurcumin and curcumin. The ranking of half-life values ($t_1/_2$) from highest to lowest is as follows: curcumin > demethoxycurcumin > bisdemethoxycurcumin.

4. Pharmacodynamics of curcuminoids

Differences in the chemical and physical properties of curcumin, demethoxycurcumin, and bisdemethoxycurcumin, resulting from variations in their chemical structures, also impact their pharmacodynamic aspects. These differences influence interactions with various receptors and enzymes, leading to pharmacological effects such as anti-inflammatory, antioxidant, anticancer, and chelating agent activities. The methoxy group in curcuminoids serves as a pharmacophore that plays a crucial role in enhancing pharmacological activities, including anti-inflammatory, antioxidant, anticancer, and chelating agent effects, as illustrated in **Figure 17** on the Qualitative Structure–Activity Relationship (QSAR) [19, 37]. From a pharmacodynamic perspective, the pharmacological response follows a potency ranking from strongest to weakest as follows: Curcumin > demethoxycurcumin > bisdemethoxycurcumin.

4.1 Antiinflammation activity of curcuminoids

One of the main mechanisms for inhibiting the inflammatory response is the inhibition of COX-2 (Cyclooxygenase-2). All types of pain and inflammation trigger the release of COX-2 mediators, as the breakdown of cell membranes containing phospholipid bilayers leads to the conversion of these components by COX-2 into various other inflammatory mediators. Curcuminoids exhibit COX-2 inhibitory activity due to their structural similarity to celecoxib, the first prototype of selective

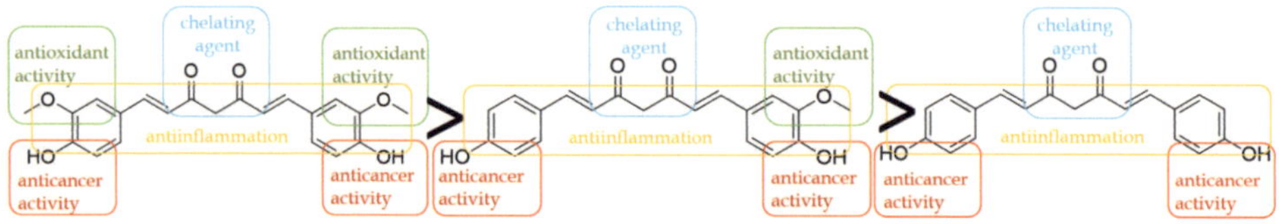

Figure 17.
Qualitative structure–activity relationship of curcuminoids.

COX-2 anti-inflammatory drugs, as well as newer-generation drugs such as etoricoxib, as shown in **Figure 18**. Curcuminoids selectively inhibit COX-2 because they possess the same pharmacophore as selective COX-2 inhibitors, including a V-shape structure, two benzoic rings, a hydrogen bond acceptor (HBA), and a hydrogen bond donor (HBD) [38, 39].

Inflammatory mediators in various diseases follow different regulatory pathways; however, COX-2 is a common pathway present in most inflammatory cases. One of the advantages of curcumin is its ability to inhibit not only the COX-2 pathway but also other inflammatory pathways, such as the Interleukin family (IL), Tumor Necrosis Factor-alpha (TNF-α), Inducible Nitric Oxide Synthase (iNOS), Macrophage Migration Inhibitory Factor (MIF), and others. For example, in Inflammatory Bowel Disease (IBD), key inflammatory mediators include the Interleukin family (IL-1, IL-6, IL-8) and Tumor Necrosis Factor-alpha (TNF-α) [40]. A comprehensive illustration of inflammatory mediators involved in specific diseases that can be inhibited by curcuminoids is presented in **Figure 19**.

The anti-inflammatory activity of curcumin is stronger compared to bisdemethoxycurcumin. The loss of two methoxy groups reduces the number of hydrogen bond acceptors, as the oxygen atom in the methoxy group acts as a hydrogen bond acceptor. This feature is one of the pharmacophores involved in inhibiting inflammatory mediators such as COX-2 [6].

4.2 Anticancer activity of curcuminoid

Curcuminoids exhibit anticancer activity at various stages of cancer cell growth inhibition. It begins with normal cells experiencing DNA damage due to exposure to physical, chemical, and biological agents, which have the potential to transform into cancer cells. At the preventive stage, curcuminoids inhibit cell growth and induce cell cycle arrest to facilitate DNA repair by increasing the activity of guardian genes such

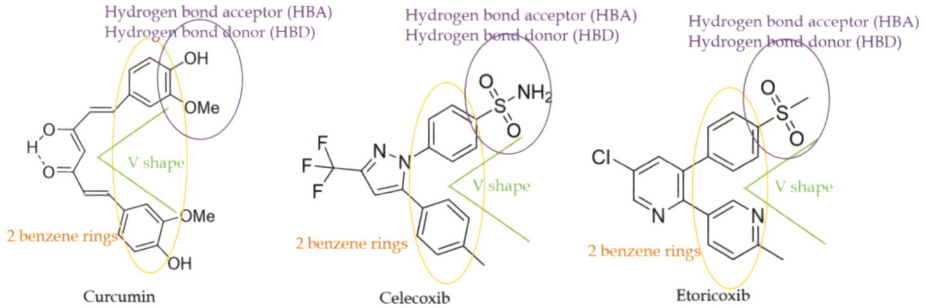

Figure 18.
Structural similarity of curcumin with COX-2 selective inhibitor drugs.

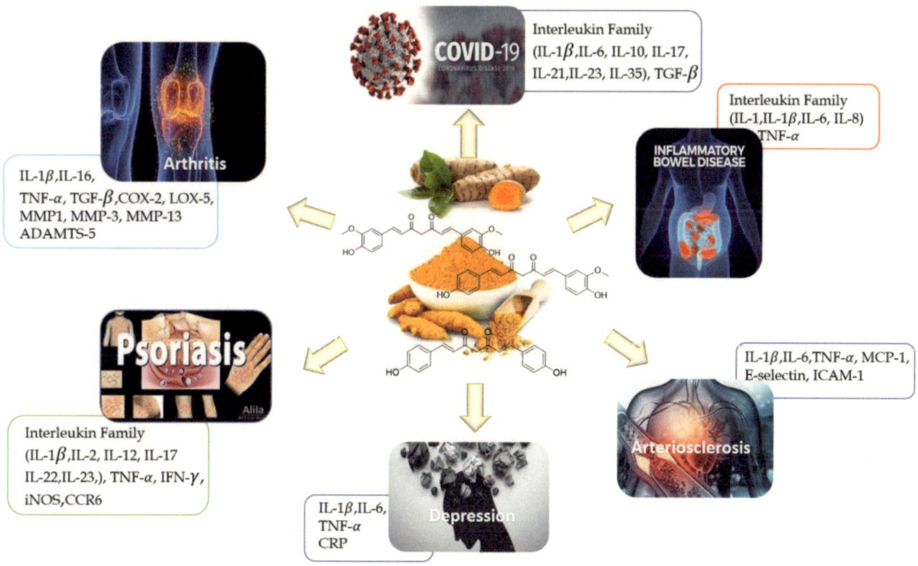

Figure 19.
Effect of curcuminoids on inflammatory bowel disease, arthritis, psoriasis, depression, and atherosclerosis.

as p53, p21, and p16, while decreasing the activity of Cyclin D1 and Cyclin E [3, 41]. If the DNA damage is too severe and cannot be repaired, curcuminoids enhance pro-apoptotic mediators such as BAX and BAK while reducing anti-apoptotic mediators such as BCL-2, BCL-xL, NF-κB, P-Akt, and mTOR [3, 41].

Apoptosis is a programmed cell death process that does not generate inflammatory mediators; if the damaged cells are not eliminated, they may continue to grow as cancer cells. Additionally, curcuminoids enhance autophagy to accelerate apoptosis by

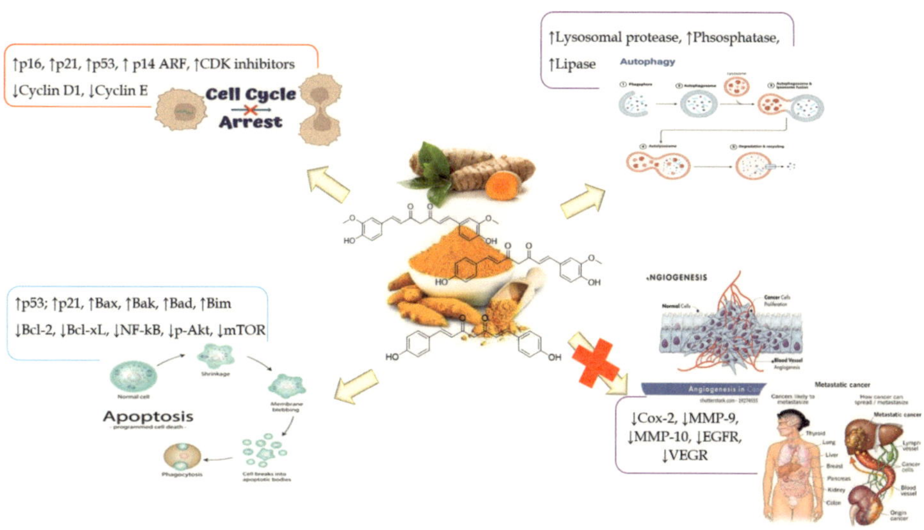

Figure 20.
Anticancer activity of curcuminoid.

increasing lysosomal proteases and proteolytic enzymes such as caspases through intrinsic (Caspase-9, Caspase-3, Caspase-6, Caspase-7) and extrinsic (Caspase-8) pathways.

At the curative stage, curcuminoids exhibit anti-angiogenesis and anti-metastasis activities. Angiogenesis is the process of forming new blood vessels from pre-existing ones, enabling cancer cells to grow more massively and aggressively due to increased nutrient and oxygen supply. Metastasis refers to the spread of cancer cells from the primary tumor to other parts of the body via the bloodstream (hematogenous), lymphatic system, or direct invasion into surrounding tissues. The mechanism by which curcuminoids inhibit angiogenesis and metastasis involves suppressing mediators such as COX-2, MMP-9, MMP-10, and VEGF [3, 41]. The anticancer activity of curcuminoids is further illustrated in **Figure 20**.

All curcuminoids contain phenolic OH groups, making them inherently active as anticancer agents. However, the anticancer activity of curcumin, both in the preventive and curative stages, is stronger due to the presence of methoxy groups, which enhance its antioxidant and chelating agent properties.

5. Conclusion

Curcuminoids are major phytochemicals widely isolated from various species of Curcuma sp. The variation in curcuminoid content among different Curcuma sp. species results in differing therapeutic effects, as curcuminoids consist of three main compounds: curcumin, demethoxycurcumin, and bisdemethoxycurcumin. The presence or absence of methoxy groups in curcuminoids alters their chemical and physical properties, which in turn affects their pharmacokinetic and pharmacodynamic profiles. The methoxy group plays a crucial role in enhancing antioxidant, anticancer, anti-inflammatory, and chelating activities. However, its presence negatively impacts pharmacokinetic properties, such as reducing gastrointestinal (GIT) absorption due to classification in BCS Class IV. Therefore, when formulating curcumin, careful consideration must be given to the drug delivery system to enhance its solubility, and permeability enhancers should be added to improve its bioavailability.

Acknowledgements

This book chapter was partially funded by Universitas Negeri Malang (Faculty Decentralization Scheme) in the grant year 2023 (Letter: 21.2.52/UN32/KP/2025).

Conflict of interest

Authors declare no conflict of interest.

Author details

Galih Satrio Putra[1*], Muhammad Ainur Hasan[1], Melanny Ika Sulistyowaty[2], Farida Anwari[3] and Dini Kesuma[4]

1 Department of Chemistry, Faculty of Mathematics and Natural Sciences, State University of Malang, Malang, Indonesia

2 Department of Pharmaceutical Sciences, Faculty of Pharmacy, Universitas Airlangga, Surabaya, Indonesia

3 Medical Laboratory Science, University of Anwar Medika, Sidoarjo, Indonesia

4 Department of Pharmaceutical Chemistry, Faculty of Pharmacy, University of Surabaya, Surabaya, Indonesia

*Address all correspondence to: galih.satrio.fmipa@um.ac.id

References

[1] Rodrigues JL, Prather KLJ, Kluskens LD, Rodrigues LR. Heterologous production of curcuminoids. Microbiology and Molecular Biology Reviews. 2015;**79**(1):39-60. DOI: 10.1128/MMBR.00031-14

[2] Banerjee A, Kotal R, Singh S, Sinha S, Mukherjee S, Seal A, et al. Identification and characterization of genes in curcuminoid pathway of Curcuma zedoaria roscoe. Current Pharmaceutical Biotechnology. 2018;**19**(10):846-854. DOI: 10.2174/1389201019666181008112244

[3] Aggarwal BB, Surh YJ, Shishodia S, editor. The Molecular Targets and Therapeutic Uses of Curcumin in Health and Disease. New York: Springer; 2007. DOI: 10.1007/978-0-387-46401-5

[4] Sulistyowaty MI, Fajrin FA, Pratama MRF, Setyawan D, Indrianingsih AW, Putra GS, et al. Anti-inflammatory potential of curcuma heyneana: An in vitro and in silico investigation. Pharmacia. 2024;**71**:1-11. DOI: 10.3897/pharmacia.71.e120886

[5] McMurry J. Organic Chemistry. 10th ed. Houston: OpenStax; 2022

[6] Clayden J, Greeves N, Warren S. Organic Chemistry. 2nd ed. Oxford: Oxford University Press; 2012

[7] Solomons TWG, Fryhle CB, Snyder SA. Organic Chemistry. 12th ed. Hoboken: Wiley; 2016

[8] Pires DE, Blundell TL, Ascher DB. pkCSM: Predicting small-molecule pharmacokinetic and toxicity properties using graph-based signatures. Journal of Medicinal Chemistry. 2015;**58**(9):4066-4072. DOI: 10.1021/acs.jmedchem.5b00104

[9] Skoog DA, West DM, Holler FJ, Crouch SR. Fundamentals of Analytical Chemistry. 10th ed. Boston: Cengage Learning; 2014

[10] Putra GS, Sulistyowaty MI, Anwari F, Syahrani A. Prediction Absorption and Biopharmaceutical Classification System (Bcs) for New Chemical Substances through in-Silico Study. Malang: Future Science Press; 2024

[11] Daina A, Michielin O, Zoete V. SwissADME: A free web tool to evaluate pharmacokinetics, drug-likeness and medicinal chemistry friendliness of small molecules. Scientific Reports. 2017;7:1-13. DOI: 10.1038/srep42717

[12] Daina A, Michielin O, Zoete V. iLOGP: A simple, robust, and efficient description of n-octanol/water partition coefficient for drug design using the GB/SA approach. Journal of Chemical Information and Modeling. 2014;**54**(12):3284-3301. DOI: 10.1021/ci500467k

[13] Ciucă MD, Racoviță RC. Curcumin: Overview of extraction methods, health benefits, and encapsulation and delivery using microemulsions and Nanoemulsions. International Journal of Molecular Sciences. 2023;**24**(10):8874. DOI: 10.3390/ijms24108874

[14] Drug Bank. Curcumin (DB11672). Drug Bank Online. [Internet]. Available from: https://go.drugbank.com/drugs/DB11672 [Accessed: March 7, 2025]

[15] National Center for Biotechnology Information (NCBI). PubChem Compound Summary for CID

969516, Curcumin. PubChem Database. [Internet]. Available from: https://pubchem.ncbi.nlm.nih.gov/compound/969516 [Accessed: March 7, 2025]

[16] National Center for Biotechnology Information (NCBI). PubChem Compound Summary for CID 5315472, Bisdemethoxycurcumin. PubChem Database. [Internet]. Available from: https://pubchem.ncbi.nlm.nih.gov/compound/5315472 [Accessed: March 8, 2025]

[17] Priyadarsini KI. The chemistry of curcumin: From extraction to therapeutic agent. Molecules. 2014;**19**(12):20091-20112. DOI: 10.3390/molecules191220091

[18] Urošević M, Nikolić L, Gajić I, Nikolić V, Dinić A, Miljković V. Curcumin: Biological activities and modern pharmaceutical forms. Antibiotics. 2022;**11**(2):135. DOI: 10.3390/antibiotics11020135

[19] Prasad S, DuBourdieu D, Srivastava A, Kumar P, Lall R. Metal–curcumin complexes in therapeutics: An approach to enhance pharmacological effects of curcumin. International Journal of Molecular Sciences. 2021;**22**(13):7094. DOI: 10.3390/ijms22137094

[20] Warren S, Wyatt P. Organic Synthesis: The Disconnection Approach. 2nd ed. Chichester: UK: Wiley; 2008

[21] Warren S, Wyatt P. Organic Synthesis: Strategy and Control. Chichester, UK: Wiley; 2007

[22] Pan X, Wang H, Li C, Zhang JZH, Ji C. MolGpka: A web server for small molecule pKa prediction using a graph-convolutional neural network. Journal of Chemical Information and Modeling. 2021;**61**(7):3159-3165. DOI: 10.1021/acs.jcim.1c00075

[23] Sinko PJ, Singh Y. Martin's Physical Pharmacy and Pharmaceutical Sciences. 8th ed. Philadelphia: Wolters Kluwer; 2023

[24] Ku MS. Use of the biopharmaceutical classification system in early drug development. The AAPS Journal. 2008;**10**(1):208-212. DOI: 10.1208/s12248-008-9020-0

[25] Samineni R, Chimakurthy J, Konidala S. Emerging role of biopharmaceutical classification and biopharmaceutical drug disposition system in dosage form development: A systematic review. Turkish Journal of Pharmaceutical Sciences. 2022;**19**(6):706-713. DOI: 10.4274/tjps.galenos.2021.73554

[26] Zhang W, Tan TM, Lim LY. Impact of curcumin-induced changes in P-glycoprotein and CYP3A expression on the pharmacokinetics of peroral celiprolol and midazolam in rats. Drug Metabolism and Disposition. 2007;**35**(1):110-115. DOI: 10.1124/dmd.106.011072

[27] Shargel L, Wu-Pong S, Yu AB. Applied Biopharmaceutics and Pharmacokinetics. 7th ed. New York: McGraw-Hill Education; 2015

[28] Buxton ILO. Pharmacokinetics: The dynamics of drug absorption, distribution, metabolism, and elimination. In: Brunton LL, Hilal-Dandan R, Knollmann BC, editors. Goodman and Gilman's: The Pharmacological Basis of Therapeutics. 13th ed. New York: McGraw-Hill Education; 2018

[29] Katzung BG, Trevor AJ. Basic and Clinical Pharmacology. 15th ed. New York: McGraw-Hill Education; 2021

[30] Singh DV, Bharti SK, Agarwal S, Roy R, Misra K. Study of interaction of

human serum albumin with curcumin by NMR and docking. Journal of Molecular Modeling. 2014;**20**(8):2365. DOI: 10.1007/s00894-014-2365-7

[31] Vukićević M, Tønnesen HH. Interaction between curcumin and human serum albumin in the presence of excipients and the effect of binding on curcumin photostability. Pharmaceutical Development and Technology. 2015;**21**: 1-9. DOI: 10.3109/10837450.2015.1016618

[32] Wang R, Wen QH, Zeng XA, Lin JW, Li J, Xu FY. Binding affinity of curcumin to bovine serum albumin enhanced by pulsed electric field pretreatment. Food Chemistry. 2022;**377**:131945. DOI: 10.1016/j.foodchem.2021.131945

[33] Drugs.com. Curcumin: Uses, Side Effects, Interactions, and Warnings. Drugs.com [Internet]; 2024. Available from: https://www.drugs.com/curcumin.html [Accessed: March 7, 2025]

[34] Bahramsoltani R, Rahimi R, Farzaei MH. Pharmacokinetic interactions of curcuminoids with conventional drugs: A review. Journal of Ethnopharmacology. 2017;**209**:1-12. DOI: 10.1016/j.jep.2017.07.022

[35] Vareed SK, Kakarala M, Ruffin MT, Crowell JA, Normolle DP, Djuric Z, et al. Pharmacokinetics of curcumin conjugate metabolites in healthy human subjects. Cancer Epidemiology, Biomarkers & Prevention. 2008;**17**(6):1411-1417. DOI: 10.1158/1055-9965.EPI-07-2693

[36] Sulistyowaty MI, Putra GS, Budiati T, Indrianingsih AW, Renawanti YW, Nofianti KA, et al. Synthesis and docking studies of the functionalized dibenzylideneacetones as promising antimalarial agents. Journal of Pharmacy and Pharmacognosy Research. 2025;**13**(2):416-430. DOI: 10.56499/jppres24.2097_13.2.416

[37] Nantasenamat C, Simeon S, Hafeez A, Prachayasittikul V, Worachartcheewan A, Songtawee N, et al. Elucidating the structure-activity relationship of curcumin and its biological activities. In: Gupta SC, Prasad S, Aggarwal BB, editors. Curcumin: Synthesis, Emerging Role in Pain Management and Health Implications. New York: Nova Biomedical; 2014. pp. 49-86

[38] Michaux C, de Leval X, Julémont F, Dogné JM, Pirotte B, Durant F. Structure-based pharmacophore of COX-2 selective inhibitors and identification of original lead compounds from 3D database searching method. European Journal of Medicinal Chemistry. 2006;**41**(12):1446-1455. DOI: 10.1016/j.ejmech.2006.07.017

[39] Sulistyowaty MI, Nugroho AE, Putra GS, Ekowati J, Budiati T. Syntheses, molecular docking study and anticancer activity examination of p-Methoxycinnamoyl hydrazides. International Journal of Pharmaceutical and Clinical Research. 2016;**8**(6):623-627

[40] Peng Y, Ao M, Dong B, Jiang Y, Yu L, Chen Z, et al. Anti-inflammatory effects of curcumin in the inflammatory diseases: Status, limitations and countermeasures. Drug Design, Development and Therapy. 2021;**15**:4503-4525. DOI: 10.2147/DDDT.S327378

[41] Wilken R, Veena MS, Wang MB, Srivatsan ES. Curcumin: A review of anti-cancer properties and therapeutic activity in head and neck squamous cell carcinoma. Molecular Cancer. 2011;**10**:12. DOI: 10.1186/1476-4598-10-12

Chapter 3

Role of Curcumin to Prevent (Thrombotic) Complications of Viral (COVID) Infections

Kirti S. Pawar, Rajnandini S. Pawar, Samragni S. Pawar and Satheesh K. Pawar

Abstract

Curcumin, the bioactive ingredient of *Curcuma longa* (turmeric) has a wide range of therapeutic effects that make it an excellent candidate for use as adjuvant therapy in the treatment of patients with COVID or any viral pneumonia. Curcumin has potential antiviral effects, including protein binding affinity toward SARS-CoV-2 proteins. Preclinical studies have shown that curcumin effectively inhibits viral infection, alleviates the severity of lung injury by offsetting the cytokine storm, and inhibits subsequent fibrosis. Curcumin inhibits thrombin and FXa and reduces blood viscosity; it could therefore alleviate COVID or any post-viral thrombotic complications viz. pulmonary fibrosis, stroke, myocardial infarction, avascular necrosis of bone, and thereby increase survival benefits.

Keywords: COVID pneumonia, curcumin, bioperine, avascular necrosis of bone, stroke, myocardial infarction

1. Introduction

COVID-19 shook the body, mind, and soul of almost every individual on this earth. Life changed enormously after the COVID-19 pandemic. It is never being the same as before. The incidence of post-COVID complications in the form of thrombotic events viz. Deep vein thrombosis, pulmonary embolism, heart attacks, stroke, and avascular necrosis of hip, is rising across the world [1].

COVID-19 treatment protocol included different drugs, each one with peculiar action hitting different targets in the pathophysiology of COVID-19 disease. Viz. 1. Antimicrobials: Antibiotics, Antivirals, Anthelmintics (to reduce the viral load): Doxycycline, Remdesivir, Favipiravir, Oseltamivir, Ivermectin. 2. Anti-inflammatory medications (to reduce the effect of cytokine storm): Hydroxychloroquine, Tocilizumab, Itolizumab. 3. Blood thinners (to prevent COVID coagulopathy and thromboembolic complications): unfractionated heparin, low molecular weight heparin. 4. Antiplatelet agent (to prevent thromboembolic complications): Aspirin. 5. Steroids as anti-inflammatory and immunosuppressant drugs (to reduce the intensity of cytokine storm and lung fibrosis): Methylprednisolone, dexamethasone. 6. Nutritional supplements (to boost immunity): Zinc, Vitamin C. Each of these drugs had its own merits and demerits and post-COVID complications were expected.

If we dip into the ocean of ancient medicines, there is one medicine, which incorporates most of the properties of drugs being used in COVID-19 treatment, named curcumin, a natural phytochemical and a blood-thinning herb [2]. Harvard College laboratory scientists, Vogel and Pelletier, from the rhizomes of *Curcuma longa* (turmeric) first discovered Curcumin about two centuries ago [3].

The therapeutic use of "*Curcuma*" has been recorded since many years [4, 5].

Curcumin played a pivotal role as an adjuvant drug in the treatment of COVID-19 due to the following reasons:

1. Studies indicate that curcumin has potential antiviral protein binding affinity toward SARS-CoV-2 proteins.

2. Curcumin exhibits a wide range of therapeutic properties including anti-inflammatory [6], antioxidant, antibacterial, antiviral, antifungal, anti-thrombotic, anti-proliferative, hypoglycemic, anticarcinogenic, neuroprotective, and cardio-protective properties [2, 7].

3. Curcumin's pleiotropic activities emanate from its ability to modulate numerous signaling molecules such as pro-inflammatory cytokines, apoptotic proteins, NF-κB, cyclooxygenase-2, 5-LOX, STAT3, C-reactive protein, prostaglandin E_2, prostate-specific antigen, adhesion molecules, phosphorylase kinase, transforming growth factor-β, triglyceride, ET-1, creatinine, HO-1, AST, and ALT in human participants [8].

4. Curcumin possesses anti-thrombotic activities by inhibiting thrombin and FXa. It has been proven to be effective in reducing the viscosity of blood and can increase survival rates [2, 9].

5. Preclinical studies demonstrate that curcumin can inhibit viral infection, reduce the severity of lung injury by preventing the cytokine storm, and inhibit subsequent fibrosis [10].

6. Curcuminoids have been approved as "Generally Recognized As Safe" (GRAS) and have good tolerability and safety profiles [11]. Its use in emergency as well as in the long run seems to be beneficial, with the least side effects compared to any presently proposed drugs in COVID-19 treatment.

Many studies have shown poor bioavailability of plain curcumin. Major reasons postulated include its poor absorption, rapid metabolism, chemical instability, and rapid systemic elimination [12, 13]. Considering this fact in acute emergency like COVID-19, we preferred oral curcumin with bioperine (bio-enhancer) over plain curcumin as bioperine increases absorption of curcumin by 2000 times [14].

2. Discussion

Efficacy of adding oral curcumin with bioperine as an adjuvant therapy in the treatment of COVID-19 disease has been assessed in double-blind, probiotic-controlled, randomized controlled study [15].

Pawar et al. [15] reported that oral curcumin with bioperine worked effectively as add-on therapy and reduced the days of remission of symptoms of COVID-19, oxygen requirement, and need for mechanical ventilation. Patients required less necessity for intravenous antiviral drugs like Inj. Remdesivir and anti-inflammatory drugs like Inj. Tocilizumab. Secondary outcomes like days of mechanical ventilation, days of hospitalization, and thromboembolic episodes in the study group were also reduced by the study drug.

For a short period of time during trial period, there was unavailability of low molecular weight heparin. However, it seems from statistical analysis that study group patients with oral curcumin with bioperine still survived better than control group. Diabetic patients also showed better results in study group than control group.

Viral infection and inflammation-induced hemoconcentration and difficulty in exchanging gases, oxygen, and carbon dioxide (a condition apparently mimicking polycythemia vera) might be the key reasons for hypoxia. Curcumin being a blood-thinning herb acted well when it was combined with antivirals and other blood thinners.

In the last week of trial, three patients from severe control group received aspirin as per physician's advice but unfortunately, none of them survived. On the contrary, severely affected patients with low platelets who received curcumin survived.

Risk factors for COVID-19 disease are age more than 60, diabetes [16, 17], hypertension [18], cardiac disease [19], chronic lung disease [20–22], cerebrovascular disease [23], chronic kidney disease [24, 25], immunosuppression [26, 27], and cancer [28] (and ironically the majority of them are on antiplatelet agents).

The use of curcumin in each of these chronic diseases is described in different studies as an effective complementary drug.

This might be the added advantage in the treatment of COVID-19 where other therapeutic agents are known to cause adverse effects on different systems of the body either immediately or in the long run, e.g. Oxygen toxicity, side effects of antivirals on liver, kidney, heparin-induced thrombocytopenia. If a drug like Curcumin, with proven benefit in all these comorbid conditions, additionally minimizes the need and side effects of other drugs and oxygen requirement in the treatment of COVID-19 disease, it might prove as a savior.

Endotoxin released by microorganisms activates macrophages and neutrophils to produce inflammatory cytokines and eicosanoids such as Thromboxane A2 [29].

Anti-inflammatory medications in the form of COX-2 inhibitors can potentially produce an imbalance in the prostaglandins produced too. Greater affinity for the COX-2 isoform likely leads to a state in which thromboxane, a proaggregatory and vaso-constructive prostaglandin produced from the COX-1 isoform, goes unchecked and might add to cardiovascular risk in patients of COVID-19 disease.

On the contrary, curcumin has an anti-inflammatory activity but it also possesses anti-thrombotic activities as it inhibits thrombin and FXa [9].

If thromboembolic complication is a part of long COVID phase, blood thinner like curcumin can save body with its blood-thinning action with least bleeding risk and can be used without coagulation profile monitoring.

Preclinical studies continuously predicted its usefulness to prevent cytokine storm [10], to prevent COVID coagulopathy [30, 31], and as an antiviral drug [32]. For the first time, our study is proving the efficacy of oral Curcumin with bioperine in human.

Oral curcumin can play a multifaceted role in the treatment of COVID-19 and can reduce absenteeism due to shortened long COVID phase and comorbidities. Antibacterial and antifungal actions of curcumin also have added advantages to lessen superinfections in COVID-19 disease process. Though it is unbelievable to accept the survival benefits of adding oral curcumin with bioperine, it is the fact, and the earliest we use it in COVID-19 patients, the fastest we are going to improve the outcome.

Another advantage of oral curcumin is no harmful side effects if stopped abruptly besides being cost-effective.

3. Conclusion

Curcumin can be a safe and natural therapeutic option to prevent and treat post-COVID thromboembolic phenomenon.

Conflict of interest

The authors declare no conflict of interest.

Author details

Kirti S. Pawar[1*], Rajnandini S. Pawar[2], Samragni S. Pawar[3] and Satheesh K. Pawar[4]

1 Siddhivinayak Health Clinic and Pain Relief Center, Baramati, India

2 HBT Medical College and Dr. R N Cooper Municipal General Hospital, Mumbai, India

3 Kasturba Medical College, Manipal, India

4 Siddhivinayak Ultrasound Research Center, Baramati, India

*Address all correspondence to: kirti.skpawar@gmail.com

References

[1] Katsoularis I, Fonseca-Rodríguez O, Farrington P, Jerndal H, Lundevaller EH, Sund M, et al. Risks of deep vein thrombosis, pulmonary embolism, and bleeding after COVID-19: Nationwide self-controlled cases series and matched cohort study. BMJ. 2022;**377**:e069590. DOI: 10.1136/bmj-2021-069590

[2] Keihanian F et al. Curcumin, hemostasis, thrombosis, and coagulation. Journal of Cellular Physiology. 2018;**233**(6):4497-4511

[3] Vogel A, Pelletier J. Examen chimique de la racine de curcuma. Journal of Pharmaceutics. 1815;**1**:289-300

[4] Loeber CC, Buechner AE. Dissertatio Inauguralis Medica de Curcuma Officinarum Ejusque Genuinis Virtutibus. In: Büchnero PAE editor. Diss Inaug Halae. Vol. 28. Halle: Halae Magdeburgicae; 1748

[5] Oppenheimer A. Turmeric (curcumin) in biliary diseases. Lancet. 1937;**229**:619-621. DOI: 10.1016/S0140-6736(00)98193-5

[6] Gupta SC, Patchva S, Aggarwal BB. Therapeutic roles of curcumin: Lessons learned from clinical trials. The AAPS Journal. 2013;**15**(1):195-218

[7] Aggarwal BB, Harikumar KB. Potential therapeutic effects of curcumin, the anti-inflammatory agent, against neurodegenerative, cardiovascular, pulmonary, metabolic, autoimmune and neoplastic diseases. The International Journal of Biochemistry & Cell Biology. 2009;**41**(1):40-59. DOI: 10.1016/j.biocel.2008.06.010

[8] Shanmugam MK et al. The multifaceted role of curcumin in cancer prevention and treatment. Molecules. 2015;**20**(2):2728-2769

[9] Kim D-C, Ku S-K, Bae J-S. Anticoagulant activities of curcumin and its derivative. BMB Reports. 2012;**45**(4):221-226. DOI: 10.5483/bmbrep.2012.45.4.221

[10] Liu Z, Ying Y. The inhibitory effect of curcumin on virus-induced cytokine storm and its potential use in the associated severe pneumonia. Frontiers in Cell and Developmental Biology. 2020;**8**:479

[11] Hewlings SJ, Kalman DS. Curcumin: A review of its' effects on human health. Food. 2017;**6**(10):92

[12] Anand P et al. Bioavailability of curcumin: Problems and promises. Molecular Pharmaceutics. 2007;**4**(6):807-818

[13] Toden S, Goel A. The holy grail of curcumin and its efficacy in various diseases: Is bioavailability truly a big concern? Journal of Restorative Medicine. 2017;**6**(1):27

[14] Han HK. The effects of black pepper on the intestinal absorption and hepatic metabolism of drugs. Expert Opinion on Drug Metabolism & Toxicology. 2011;**7**:721-729. DOI: 10.1517/17425255.2011.570332

[15] Pawar KS et al. Oral curcumin with piperine as adjuvant therapy for the treatment of COVID-19: A randomized clinical trial. Frontiers in Pharmacology. 2021;**12**:1

[16] Zhang D-w, Fu M, Gao S-H, Liu J-L. Curcumin and diabetes: A systematic review. Evidence-based Complementary

and Alternative Medicine. 2013;**2013**:1-6. DOI: 10.1155/2013/636053

[17] Poolsup N et al. Effects of curcumin on glycemic control and lipid profile in prediabetes and type 2 diabetes mellitus: A systematic review and meta-analysis. PLoS One. 2019;**14**(4):e0215840

[18] Leong X-F. The spice for hypertension: Protective role of curcuma longa. Biomedical and Pharmacology Journal. 2018;**11**(4):1829-1840

[19] Wongcharoen W, Phrommintikul A. The protective role of curcumin in cardiovascular diseases. International Journal of Cardiology. 2009;**133**(2):145-151

[20] Venkatesan N, Punithavathi D, Babu M. Protection from acute and chronic lung diseases by curcumin. In: The Molecular Targets and Therapeutic Uses of Curcumin in Health and Disease. Boston, MA: Springer; 2007. pp. 379-405

[21] Biswas S, Rahman I. Modulation of steroid activity in chronic inflammation: A novel anti-inflammatory role for curcumin. Molecular Nutrition & Food Research. 2008;**52**(9):987-994

[22] Moriyuki K et al. Curcumin inhibits the proteinase-activated receptor-2–triggered prostaglandin E2 production by suppressing cyclooxygenase-2 upregulation and Akt-dependent activation of nuclear factor-κB in human lung epithelial cells. Journal of Pharmacological Sciences. 2010;**114**(2):225-229

[23] Ovbiagele B. Potential role of curcumin in stroke prevention. Expert Review of Neurotherapeutics. 2008;**8**(8):1175-1176

[24] Ghosh SS, Gehr TWB, Ghosh S. Curcumin and chronic kidney disease (CKD): Major mode of action through stimulating endogenous intestinal alkaline phosphatase. Molecules. 2014;**19**(12):20139-20156

[25] de Almeida Alvarenga L et al. Curcumin-A promising nutritional strategy for chronic kidney disease patients. Journal of Functional Foods. 2018;**40**:715-721

[26] Sharma S et al. Resveratrol and curcumin suppress immune response through CD28/CTLA-4 and CD80 co-stimulatory pathway. Clinical & Experimental Immunology. 2007;**147**(1):155-163

[27] Mollazadeh H et al. Immune modulation by curcumin: The role of interleukin-10. Critical Reviews in Food Science and Nutrition. 2019;**59**(1):89-101

[28] Ravindran J, Prasad S, Aggarwal BB. Curcumin and cancer cells: How many ways can curry kill tumor cells selectively? The AAPS Journal. 2009;**11**(3):495-510

[29] Conti P et al. IL-1 induces throboxane-A2 (TxA2) in COVID-19 causing inflammation and micro-thrombi: Inhibitory effect of the IL-1 receptor antagonist (IL-1Ra). Journal of Biological Regulators and Homeostatic Agents. 2020;**34**:4

[30] Singh K. Potential role of curcumin against viral infections with a view on structure and pathogenesis of COVID-19. AIJR Preprints. 2020. DOI: 10.21467/preprints.213

[31] Suresh PS. Curcumin and coagulopathy in the COVID-19 era. Indian Journal of Clinical Biochemistry. 2020;**35**(4):504-505. DOI: 10.1007/s12291-020-00914-5

[32] Zahedipour F, Hosseini SA, Sathyapalan T, Majeed M, Jamialahmadi T, Al-Rasadi K, et al. Potential effects of curcumin in the treatment of COVID-19 infection. Phytotherapy Research. 2020;**34**(11):2911-2920. DOI: 10.1002/ptr.6738

Chapter 4

Potential Clinical Value of Curcumin and Its Therapeutic Benefits in Cancer and Human Health

Shimaa E. Rashad

Abstract

Scientists from all over the world have been interested in curcumin, a polyphenol that was extracted from *Curcuma longa* in 1815, because of its biological properties (such as antiviral, anti-inflammatory, antioxidant, and antimicrobial properties). Of these, its anticancer potential has been well-documented and is still being studied. Because of its strong anti-inflammatory, antioxidant, anticancer, immunomodulatory, neuroprotective, antiproliferative, and antibacterial properties, curcumin—a hydrophobic polyphenol that was extracted from the rhizome of *Curcuma longa*—is now being considered as a potential medication for the treatment of neurological conditions, such as Parkinson's disease (PD), Alzheimer's disease (AD), Huntington's disease (HD), multiple sclerosis (MS), amyotrophic lateral sclerosis (ALS), prion disease, and Alzheimer's disease. In Asia, India, and China, curcumin has long been utilized for both medical and culinary purposes. To successfully carry the active medication to brain cells, several nanocarriers have been produced, including liposomes, micelles, dendrimers, cubosome nanoparticles, polymer nanoparticles, and solid lipid nanoparticles. Target-specificity is achieved by functionalizing the surface of nanoparticles with brain-specific ligands, which should greatly increase bioavailability and lessen adverse effects. In addition to directly binding to and limiting the aggregation of amyloid's β-sheet conformations, which are a hallmark of many neurodegenerative diseases, curcumin is a pleiotropic molecule that also scavenges free radicals, chelates iron, induces antioxidant response elements, and restores the inflammatory system's homeostasis. This review aims to summarize the studies on curcumin and/or nanoparticles containing curcumin in the most common neurodegenerative diseases, highlighting the high neuroprotective potential of this nutraceutical.

Keywords: curcumin, cancer, Alzheimer's disease, amyloid, amyloid-binding, antioxidant, activator protein 1, brain derived neurotrophic factor, C-Jun N terminal kinase, heat shock proteins, misfolded proteins, neurodegeneraton, neuroinflammation, non-steroidal anti-inflammatory drugs, nuclear factor Kappa B, polyphenolic antioxidants, neurodegenerative diseases, nanoparticles, *Curcuma longa*, bioavailability

1. Introduction

The rhizome of *Curcuma longa* L., commonly known as turmeric, contains curcumin, a compound from the diarylheptanoid class of natural products (curcuminoids). Other curcuminoids, such as demethoxycurcumin and bis-demethoxycurcumin (1–6%), as well as various turmeric oils (3–7%), have also been studied [1].

Recent research has highlighted three innovative applications of turmeric (*Curcuma longa* L.): regulating gut microbiota, using curcumin-loaded exosome vesicles, and developing turmeric-derived exosome-like vesicles to overcome application limitations. Additionally, curcumin analogs and related compounds are being explored for their potential benefits [1].

Turmeric is now cultivated in regions, including South America, China, and Southeast Asia, where its high curcuminoid content is believed to contribute to its therapeutic properties. Curcumin (CUR) and its derivatives, demethoxycurcumin (DMC) and bisdemethoxycurcumin (BDMC) are linear diarylheptanoids derived from the rhizomes. Curcumin, a crystalline substance with a vibrant orange-yellow color, is commonly used as a food additive and coloring agent [2].

Curcumin is classified as a safe food ingredient under international regulations. The World Health Organization (WHO) has set the acceptable daily intake (ADI) for curcumin as a food coloring agent between 0 and 3 mg/kg [3]. The US Food and Drug Administration (USFDA) has recognized curcumin as "generally recognized as safe" (GRAS) [4]. While curcumin is well-known for its wide-ranging pharmacological properties and safety profile in both humans and animals, high doses (greater than 50,000 ppm) taken to address its low bioavailability may result in adverse effects and raise safety concerns **Figure 1** [5].

Curcumin-loaded hydrogels and nanoparticles represent innovative delivery technologies that have shown promise in improving curcumin bioavailability and enhancing its therapeutic effects. Another emerging approach is photodynamic therapy, where exposure to light enhances curcumin's anticancer properties by influencing biochemical pathways critical to tumor cell growth and survival. Studies indicate that combining curcumin with visible light irradiation at low concentrations significantly

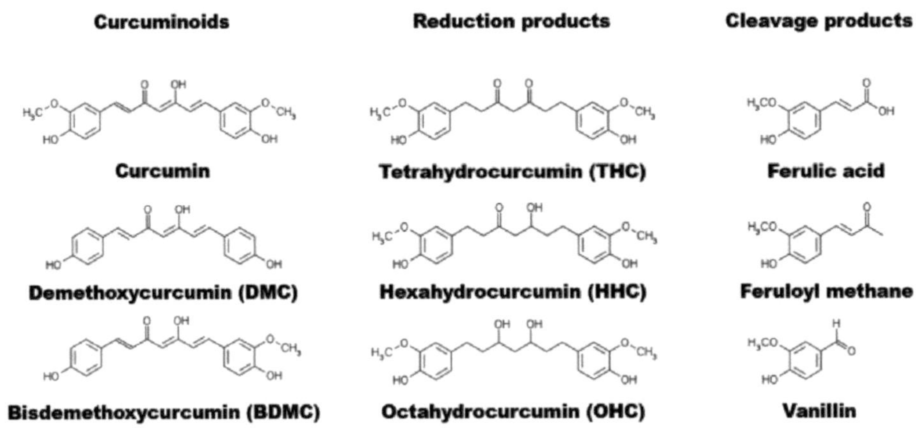

Figure 1.
Curcuminoids, curcumin metabolites (reduction), and their breakdown products (cleavage) [1]. https://www.ncbi.nlm.nih.gov/core/lw/2.0/html/tileshop_pmc/tileshop_pmc_inline.html?title=Click%20on%20image%20to%20zoom&p=PMC3&id=10281727_jfda194-211f1.jpg.

boosts its anticancer activity. However, caution must be exercised in clinical settings, as curcumin's interaction with cytochromes or drug transporters could impact the pharmacokinetics of conventional medications [6].

The rhizome of *Curcuma longa*, or turmeric, produces curcumin, a polyphenolic compound (**Figure 2**) [7, 8]. This compound, along with other precursors such as demethoxycurcumin and bis-demethoxycurcumin, undergoes a series of enzymatic modifications [9]. Curcumin, the primary active compound responsible for the medicinal properties and the vibrant yellow-orange color of turmeric, is formed through these biochemical processes (**Figure 2**) [10]. The rhizomes of the turmeric plant are the site of this biosynthetic activity, which plays a key role in the plant's defense mechanisms against infections and oxidative stress [8].

While curcumin's beneficial effects have primarily been observed in *in vitro* studies, it is crucial to recognize its limitations *in vivo* (**Figure 3**). Its rapid metabolism and poor absorption after administration can significantly reduce its bioavailability and clinical potential. Curcumin has limited intestinal absorption, is rapidly metabolized in the liver, and has poor water solubility [11]. As a result, a substantial portion of ingested curcumin may not be effectively absorbed by the body. The liver quickly breaks down curcumin into metabolites with less biological activity, limiting the amount of the active compound that reaches systemic circulation and targets [11].

To achieve therapeutic effects, large doses of curcumin are often required. Although the food and drug administration (FDA) has classified curcumin as "generally recognized as safe" (GRAS) and generally well-tolerated, high doses can lead to issues such as hepatotoxicity, gastrointestinal disturbances (including nausea, diarrhea, or stomach pain), and tolerance problems that may be difficult to manage [12, 13].

Curcumin has also been shown to affect blood coagulation. Numerous studies suggest it has anticoagulant and antiplatelet properties. Specifically, curcumin can extend prothrombin time and activated partial thromboplastin time, both of which are tests used to measure blood coagulation. These findings suggest curcumin may reduce the risk of clot formation by slowing blood coagulation [14]. Its antithrombotic effects are further supported by evidence showing curcumin inhibits platelet activation and

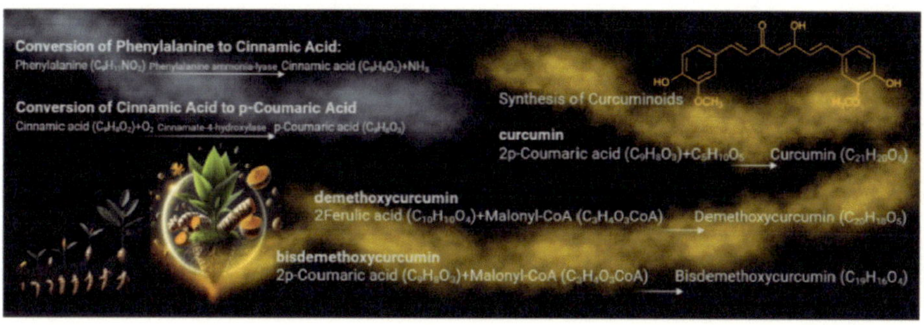

Figure 2.
The production of curcumin in the rhizomes of Curcuma longa *involves several enzymatic steps. Initially, phenylalanine is converted into cinnamic acid by phenylalanine ammonia-lyase. From cinnamic acid, p-coumaric acid, an important intermediate, is formed. Through a series of enzymatic reactions, p-coumaric acid is further transformed into the curcuminoid precursors—curcumin, demethoxycurcumin, and bis-demethoxycurcumin. Methylation and other modifications of p-coumaric acid lead to the formation of ferulic acid, which is then converted into demethoxycurcumin. These biochemical processes contribute to the plant's defense mechanisms, protecting it from infections and oxidative stress. https://www.mdpi.com/cancers/cancers-16 02580/article_deploy/html/images/cancers-16-02580-g001.png.*

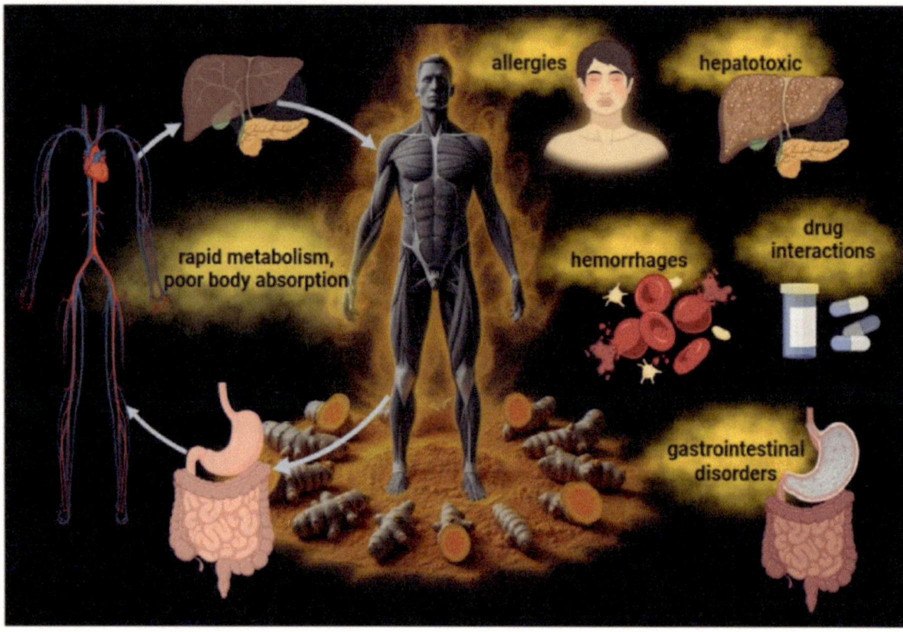

Figure 3.
There are several limitations to using curcumin as a treatment for patients due to its low bioavailability. Its poor absorption in the intestines, rapid metabolism in the liver, and low solubility in water all contribute to these challenges. To achieve therapeutic effects, high doses of curcumin are often needed, which can lead to side effects such as allergies, gastrointestinal issues, hepatotoxicity, and potential anticoagulant or antiplatelet effects. Additionally, curcumin may interact with various medications, including those for cardiovascular conditions, anti-inflammatory drugs, anticancer treatments, and antibiotics. https://www.mdpi.com/cancers/cancers-16-02580/article_deploy/html/images/cancers-16-02580-g002.png.

aggregation. Since thrombosis and atherothrombosis are significant risk factors for cardiovascular diseases, curcumin's effects may be particularly beneficial in preventing these conditions [15]. However, it is important to note that, while curcumin may function as a natural anticoagulant, its use should be carefully monitored, especially when combined with other anticoagulant medications, as this could amplify their effects and increase the risk of bleeding. Individuals currently undergoing anticoagulant therapy should consult their doctor before taking turmeric supplements or products. Additionally, curcumin may interact with certain medications, such as anti-inflammatory and anticancer drugs [16].

2. Turmeric's composition

2.1 Curcumin and its derivatives: Production, applications, and therapeutic potential

Curcumin ($C21H20O5$), also known as diferuloylmethane, is a bioactive compound extracted from the rhizomes of *Curcuma longa* (turmeric). It is structurally characterized as (1E,6E)-1,7-bis(4-hydroxy-3-methoxyphenyl)hepta-1,6-diene-3,5-dione. In addition to curcumin, two other curcuminoids, demethoxycurcumin (DMC) ($C20H18O5$) and bis-demethoxycurcumin (BDMC) ($C19H16O4$), are present in varying concentrations across different Curcuma species. These compounds are biosynthesized through a series of enzymatic reactions in the rhizomes of the plant.

Notably, the concentration of curcuminoids can vary depending on geographical location, with *C. longa* grown in regions like Pengzhou Sichuan, China, containing the highest levels of curcuminoids (40.36 mg/g) compared to other regions [17].

The antimicrobial properties of turmeric extracts have been demonstrated in several studies. For example, the growth of *S. aureus* was inhibited, and the growth of *Pseudomonas* sp., *E. faecalis*, and *L. innocua* was significantly reduced at concentrations of 0.1 and 1.0 mg TE/mL. Additionally, at a concentration of 10 mg TE/mL, all tested microorganisms, including *E. coli*, showed decreased growth. The antioxidant capacity of turmeric ethanol extract, as measured by assays such as HOSC, RDSC, and 2,2'-azino-bis(3-ethylbenzothiazoline-6-sulfonic acid (ABTS), highlighted its potential for reducing oxidative stress and supporting microbial load reduction [18]. Furthermore, the curcuminoid content of turmeric varies with geographic location, with samples from warmer climates (e.g., Southern Nepal) containing higher concentrations than those from cooler regions (e.g., Northern Nepal) [19].

In line with the standards outlined in official pharmacopeias such as the Taiwan Herbal Pharmacopoeia [20] and The Pharmacopeia of the People's Republic of China 2020 Edition [21], medicinal turmeric must contain at least 1% curcumin. However, the curcumin content of turmeric roots is typically lower than that of rhizomes, and the location of the plant must be considered for accurate dosage determination [22]. Furthermore, curcumin may break down into metabolites like ferulic acid, feruloyl methane, and vanillin in neutral to alkaline liquids [23].

3. Clinical significance of curcumin

Since its first isolation in 1870, curcumin has been used extensively in Asia as a natural coloring agent and food additive. Its first documented biological activity as an antibacterial agent was reported in 1949 [24]. Over time, research has uncovered its broad therapeutic potential, including antiviral, anti-inflammatory, anticancer, and antioxidant properties. Curcumin's therapeutic effects have been extensively studied *in vitro*, *in vivo*, and in clinical settings, showcasing its potential to treat chronic diseases.

Curcumin, along with its derivatives like Dihydrocurcumin and Tetrahydrocurcumin, offers various health benefits, including immunological regulation, cardiovascular protection, and neuroprotection. To overcome curcumin's limitations in bioavailability, including poor absorption, rapid metabolism, and quick elimination, novel strategies such as nanoparticle encapsulation, adjuvant therapy with piperine or quercetin, and the use of metformin have been explored [25, 26]. Despite the significant therapeutic promise, challenges remain in improving curcumin's bioavailability and biocompatibility [27, 28].

3.1 Antioxidant properties

Curcumin is recognized as a potent antioxidant that helps protect the body from free-radical damage. It has been shown to enhance the levels of antioxidants like superoxide dismutase (SOD) in the blood. Unlike synthetic antioxidants, which may have harmful side effects, curcumin is considered a safer alternative for reducing oxidative damage [29]. It contains functional groups, such as the 1,2-dihydroxy group, which contribute to its strong antioxidant properties. Curcumin is being researched for its potential in treating conditions like cardiovascular disease, Parkinson's disease, Alzheimer's disease, and promoting wound healing [30].

3.2 Anti-inflammatory and anti-tumor effects

Curcumin has demonstrated anti-inflammatory and anti-tumor effects through several mechanisms, including inhibition of matrix metalloproteinases, growth factors like HER-2 and epidermal growth factor receptor (EGFR), and signaling pathways such as STAT3 and NF-kB. These actions help reduce the release of inflammatory mediators and promote apoptosis in tumor cells. Curcumin has also been shown to enhance wound healing by modulating inflammatory cell death, which accelerates the resolution of inflammation [31, 32].

3.3 Molecular targets of curcumin

Curcumin shows promise in preventing and treating various diseases by modulating the expression of key proteins involved in disease progression. For example, in the case of colorectal cancer, curcumin may influence signaling pathways associated with susceptibility genes. Additionally, curcumin has been investigated for its potential to prevent skin diseases by modulating the expression of protein kinase C epsilon (PKCε) [33–35].

3.4 Prevention of cataracts and diabetes-related nephropathy

Curcumin has been studied for its potential to prevent cataracts associated with diabetes. Research has also explored its role in managing diabetic nephropathy (DN) symptoms, offering a therapeutic option for patients recovering from this condition [36, 37]. Studies have shown that curcumin can influence plasma asprosin levels, insulin resistance, and glucose metabolism in diabetic rats, highlighting its antidiabetic properties [38, 39].

3.5 Neuroprotective effects

Curcumin has demonstrated neuroprotective effects in age-related neurodegenerative diseases (NDs) by reducing cellular inflammation and oxidative stress. It has been shown to reduce motor and cognitive decline in aging individuals and animal models of Alzheimer's disease (AD) [40, 41]. Curcumin's ability to modulate the expression of CISD2, a protein associated with mitochondrial dysfunction, contributes to its neuroprotective properties [42–45].

4. Medicinal use of curcumin

Curcumin has proven anticancer properties, inhibiting tumor growth and metastasis by blocking key signaling pathways involved in cancer progression. It suppresses transcription factors and downstream gene products, including c-myc, COX-2, NOS, Cyclin D1, TNF-α, and interleukins. Curcumin has been shown to significantly affect prostate cancer cells while having minimal effects on normal human prostate epithelial cells [46, 47].

In summary, curcumin's therapeutic potential spans a wide range of chronic diseases, and ongoing research is critical to fully understanding its mechanisms of action and improving its clinical application **Table 1**.

Effects	Models	Mechanism of action	Finding
Chemopreventive	Sprague-Dawley rats	Enhances the characteristics of the GST enzyme.	The expression of rGST8-8, an α-class GST isozyme involved in protecting against lipid peroxidation products, is particularly influenced by curcumin.
	Bovine aortic endothelial cells	Increasing HO-1 mRNA, protein expression, and overall properties.	This research explores how different doses of curcumin affect endothelial heme oxygenase activity and HO-1 protein expression.
Anti-carcinogenesis	BP-induced lung tumor in mice	It reduces LPO and ROS levels while improving the activity of SOD and GST enzymes.	The findings show that both curcumin and quercetin provide protection to mice against lung carcinogenesis induced by benzo(a)pyrene.
	CoCl2-induced hypoxia in HCC		
Anti-cytotoxic	MG-induced cell death in human hepatoma G2 cells	Hypoxia-induced reduction in HIF-1α protein suppresses cell migration, invasion, and proliferation, and modifies epithelial-mesenchymal transition (EMT).	Curcumin significantly reduces ROS formation, which triggers cytochrome c release, caspase activation, and subsequent apoptotic changes.
	PhIP-induced cytotoxicity in breast epithelial cells	Curcumin also minimizes oxidative stress (OS) and prevents apoptotic biochemical changes, including PARP cleavage, caspase-3 activation, and cytochrome c release.	It notably decreases ROS production, as well as PhIP-induced DNA adduct formation and double-strand breaks.
Chemo-protective	TAA-induced liver inflammation and fibrosis in rats	It reduces ROS production, inhibits DNA adducts and double-strand breaks, and promotes the expression of genes involved in DNA repair and antioxidant defense.	This study examines curcumin's hepatoprotective effects on hepatocellular carcinoma through autophagic and apoptotic pathways.
	Hemin-induced cytotoxicity in rat neurons.	Additionally, curcumin suppresses ROS generation, reduces the GSH/GSSG ratio, and increases the levels of GR, GST, and SOD enzymes. It also raises HO-1 levels and enhances Nrf2 translocation to the nucleus, which collectively contribute to reduced cell death.	Pre-treatment with curcumin increases glutathione (GSH) and HO-1 expression, demonstrating its protective ability against toxicity induced by hemin.
Cell cycle arrest	Breast cancer MCF-7 cells	Curcumin inhibits cyclin B1, Cdc2, and NF-κB by decreasing the interaction between pIκB and NF-κB.	
Anti-tumorigenesis	CML-derived K562 cells, xenograft mouse	Derivatives elevate ROS levels, compete with coenzymes for binding to relevant ROS metabolic enzymes, and hinder their function.	Curcumin inhibits cyclin B1 and Cdc2, preventing colony formation in MCF-7 wt cells and causing cell cycle arrest at the G2/M phase.

Effects	Models	Mechanism of action	Finding
Autophagy and apoptosis	lymphoma HuT-78 cells		The overproduction of ROS in curcumin compounds may lead to the development of low-side-effect anticancer drugs.
Chemosensitization	Glioblastoma	It generates ROS, inhibits NF-κB, accumulates the autophagy marker LC3-I, degrades Hsp90 to disrupt IKK and beclin-1 integrity, and blocks c-FLIP, Bcl-xL, cIAP, and XIAP. Through caspase-3 cleavage, key substrates are degraded, leading to apoptosis.	The results also show that DMC significantly reduces cell growth *in vitro* and enhances glutamine synthetase (GSC) apoptosis prior to TMZ treatment.
Autophagy	Colon cancer HCT116 cells	JAK/STAT3 pathway inactivation, and increased ROS production, DMC enhances TMZ-induced apoptosis.	Additionally, ROS plays a key role in curcumin-induced autophagic cell death.

Table 1.
The cancer-preventive effects of curcumin are described [48].

4.1 Curcumin displays notable antiproliferative properties and anticancer potential

Extensive research, including completed and ongoing studies, aims to address its limitations. Curcumin, either alone or in combination with other treatments, could play a transformative role in cancer therapy [49, 50]. Its antiproliferative effects are primarily observed through its influence on NF-κB, cell cycle regulation, tubulin, proteasomes, EGFRs, caspases, and STATs. Additionally, a list of compounds with the most potent antiproliferative activity, such as CBA-pR, has been identified **Table 2** and **Figure 4**.

4.2 Anti-metastatic properties of curcumin

Metastasis is the process through which cancer cells spread from the primary tumor to other parts of the body, significantly affecting patient prognosis and survival rates. The ability of tumor cells to disseminate contributes to their destructive

Mechanism of action
Regulation of Th17/Treg balance
Modulation of microbial diversity and abundance
Improvement of gut microbiota composition
Influence on immune modulation
Restoration of gut flora balance
Enhancement of cytarabine response in acute myeloid leukemia
Indirect influence on neuroprotection through modulation of signaling pathways
Modulation of intestinal barrier function

Table 2.
Curcumin's mechanisms of action [51].

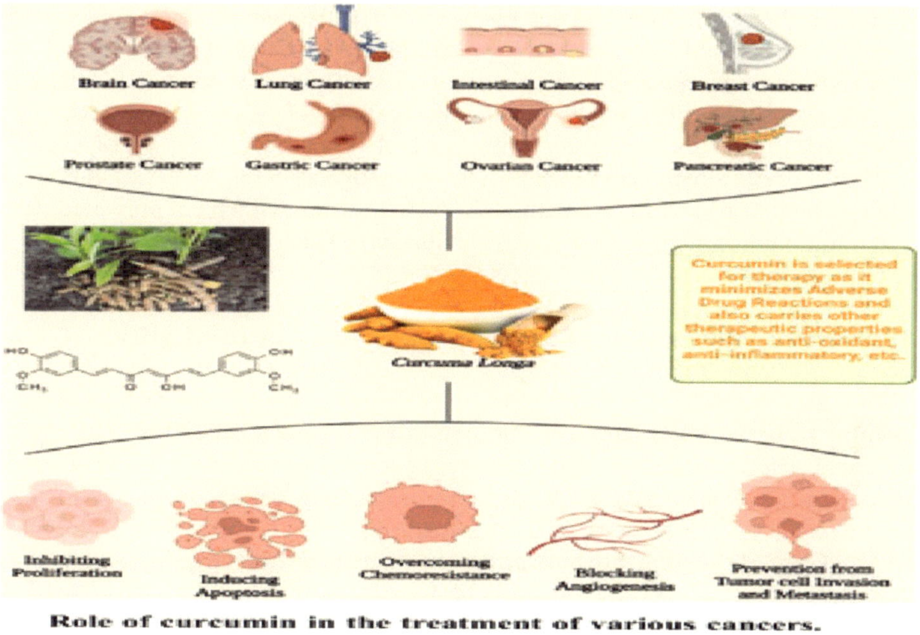

Figure 4.
Curcumin's role in treating different types of cancer [50].

potential [52]. Revascularization plays a critical role in cancer progression, facilitating the spread and growth of malignant cells at distant sites [53]. Curcumin, a polyphenolic compound derived from *Curcuma longa*, has demonstrated immunosuppressive properties, as highlighted in recent studies [54]. Experiments involving U-2 OS and MG-63 osteosarcoma cell lines treated with DK1 have further evaluated curcumin's potential as an anti-metastatic agent [55].

4.3 Curcumin and apoptosis

Curcumin has been shown to modulate key molecular pathways involved in apoptosis, such as the PI3K/Akt pathway, which is often dysregulated in various cancers, including glioblastoma, breast, prostate, and head and neck cancers. The Ras/Raf/MAPK and PI3K/Akt/mTOR pathways, both frequently altered in malignancies, not only drive cancer cell proliferation independently but also interact with other regulatory networks, such as the β-catenin/Wnt, Notch, and p53-mediated apoptosis pathways [56]. Studies on colorectal cancer cells (HCT-116) have revealed concentration-dependent suppression of cell survival, with curcumin interacting with tumor suppressors and oncogenes like TP53, Bax, Wnt-1, and CTNNB1 [57]. Notably, the synergistic effect of curcumin in combination with resveratrol has been observed in modulating multiple oncogenic signaling pathways [58]. Additionally, curcumin is known to reduce oxidative stress and induce autophagy, potentially enhancing cellular health and organismal well-being [58].

4.4 Curcumin and angiogenesis inhibition

Curcumin has been found to influence angiogenesis, a key process in tumor progression. Research on human umbilical vein endothelial cells (HUVECs) has shown that oxidized low-density lipoprotein (ox-LDL) induces cellular damage, increasing cell proliferation, migration, and angiogenesis [59]. Curcumin treatment counteracts these effects by inhibiting the Wnt/β-catenin pathway, which plays a crucial role in angiogenic processes [60]. Furthermore, the administration of SKL2001, a β-catenin agonist, has been shown to mitigate the inhibitory effects of curcumin on angiogenesis [61]. Additionally, curcumin enhances hypomethylation in response to oxidative stress, which may further regulate angiogenesis-related genes. A novel finding is curcumin's role in increasing HLA-G expression, which not only modulates the immune environment for invasive trophoblasts but also positively influences angiogenesis [62].

4.5 Curcumin's influence on cellular senescence and telomere integrity

Telomeres, specialized DNA structures at chromosome ends, prevent genomic instability by protecting against recombination and degradation [63]. Telomere shortening occurs naturally due to replication and oxidative damage, particularly through reactive oxygen species (ROS) in fibroblast cells [64, 65]. Exposure to radiation and oxidative stress triggers a DNA damage response, contributing to telomere attrition. Current research into anticancer strategies targeting telomerase and cellular senescence is still developing. Stilbene-based compounds have been identified as promising agents that can induce senescence and inhibit telomerase activity in cancer cells, providing potential therapeutic avenues for targeting telomere dynamics [66].

5. Curcumin and the intestinal microbiota

Despite its low systemic bioavailability, curcumin exerts profound effects on gut microbiota composition, promoting the growth of beneficial bacteria such as Bifidobacterial and Lactobacilli while suppressing pathogenic strains [43]. The human gut microbiome consists of diverse microorganisms, including bacteria, fungi, and viruses, with Firmicutes and Bacteroidetes representing the dominant phyla. Curcumin influences metabolic and inflammatory pathways through its effects on gut microbial metabolites, particularly those associated with energy production and fatty acid metabolism [44]. These findings highlight curcumin's potential in developing novel therapeutic strategies for neurodegenerative diseases, as gut dysbiosis has been linked to altered endocrine signaling and metabolic dysfunction [67].

5.1 Gut microbiota and glucose regulation

Curcumin plays a role in regulating glucose metabolism, particularly in conditions like metabolic syndrome and type 2 diabetes [68]. Despite its limited bioavailability, curcumin interacts with gut microbiota, helping restore eubiotic balance, which is crucial for maintaining glycemic homeostasis. Supplementation with curcumin has demonstrated beneficial effects on intestinal microbial composition, enhancing gut health through its immunomodulatory, neuroprotective, and anti-inflammatory properties [69]. However, challenges remain in optimizing curcumin's bioavailability and ensuring its safety for therapeutic applications [70].

5.2 Effects on intestinal barrier function

The intestinal barrier prevents harmful substances from penetrating healthy colonic tissue, and its disruption is linked to chronic inflammation, a major risk factor for colon cancer and metabolic disorders such as atherosclerosis and diabetes. Curcumin has been shown to enhance intestinal barrier integrity, making it a potential candidate for preventing and treating gastrointestinal disorders [71].

5.3 Curcumin and intestinal inflammation

Obesity-related systemic inflammation is a major contributor to metabolic diseases. Curcumin, a bioactive compound in turmeric, possesses anti-inflammatory properties that may reduce obesity-induced inflammation. Research indicates that curcumin modulates gut microbiota composition, promoting beneficial microbial populations while reducing harmful strains [72]. These microbial shifts are associated with a decline in microbial diversity and alterations in pathways involved in intestinal inflammation. Mechanistically, curcumin enhances gut barrier function by regulating tight junction proteins and mitigating inflammation *via* the suppression of p38 MAPK and myosin light chain kinase activation [48]. Additionally, curcumin influences neuroprotection by interacting with gut microbiota through NF-kB and AP-1 signaling pathways. In models of Parkinson's disease, curcumin has been shown to reduce neuroinflammation and improve motor impairments by modulating the gut microbiota-metabolite axis **Figure 5** [33].

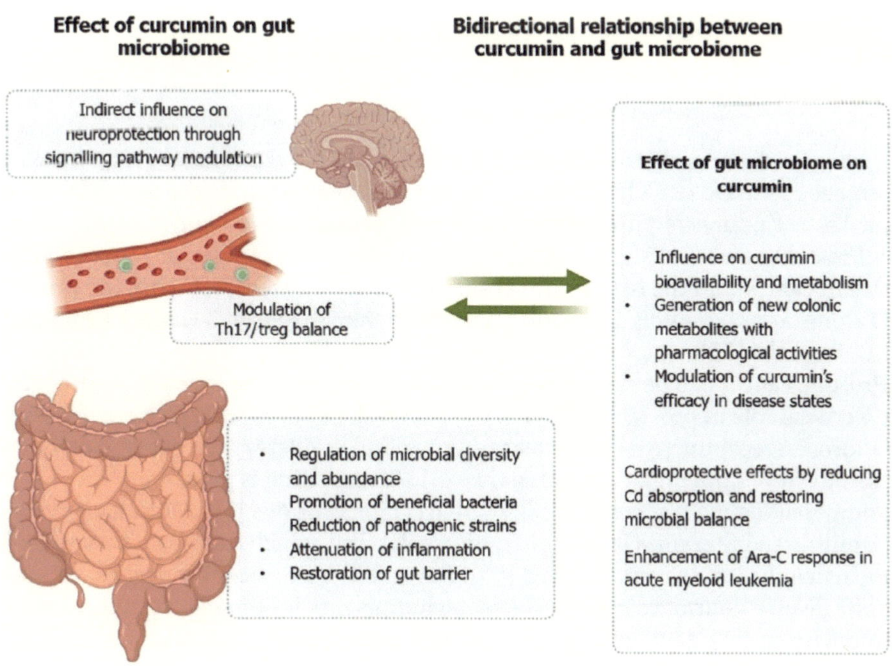

Figure 5.
Curcumin's impact on the gut microbiota [51].

6. Curcumin's impact on cancer

6.1 Agents that fight cancer

Curcumin is recognized for its medicinal potential due to its antimicrobial, antioxidant, and anti-inflammatory properties. Its ability to regulate various cellular processes and signaling pathways makes it a promising therapeutic agent for multiple human diseases, including cancer, cardiovascular conditions, and neurodegenerative disorders. Although curcumin has limited bioavailability, advancements in drug delivery methods—such as liposomal formulations and nanoparticles—have enhanced its solubility and systemic absorption, improving its therapeutic potential.

The antioxidant properties of curcumin play a crucial role in preventing and managing chronic inflammatory diseases, which are often linked to severe conditions like cancer, as well as neurological disorders such as Parkinson's and Alzheimer's disease [73]. Since its initial extraction from *Curcuma longa*, curcumin has been widely studied for its broad therapeutic applications. It exhibits diverse biological activities, including anti-inflammatory, antioxidant, anticancer, anti-asthmatic, anti-arthritic, neuroprotective, antidiabetic, anti-obesity, wound healing, hepatoprotective, and skin-regenerative effects. Chemically, curcumin is known as 1,7-bis(4-hydroxy-3-methoxyphenyl)-1,6-heptadiene-3,5-dione, or diferuloylmethane.

Numerous clinical trials have explored curcumin's effectiveness in these areas, assessing its influence on key molecular pathways. During inflammation, factors such as AKT, ROS, NF-κB, AP-1, cytokines, and COX-2 contribute to tumor development by promoting a pro-inflammatory environment [74, 75]. Curcumin has been shown to modulate these pathways, making it a valuable candidate for cancer treatment. Its role in various cancer therapies is illustrated in **Figure 6**.

6.2 Prostate cancer

Turmeric-derived phytocompounds have demonstrated potential as inhibitors of ribosomal S6 kinase (RSK), which may be beneficial for prostate cancer (PCa) treatment. These findings require further validation through *in vitro* and *in vivo* studies [76]. Prostate cancer is a significant global health concern, ranking as the second most prevalent cancer and the fifth leading cause of cancer-related deaths among men. In 2020 alone, approximately 1.4 million new cases were diagnosed, leading to around 500,000 deaths [77].

Prostate cancer can be categorized based on its androgen sensitivity. Androgens play a crucial role in prostate epithelial cell survival and proliferation by activating the androgen receptor (AR), a nuclear receptor that regulates gene expression related to prostate development and maintenance [3]. AR signaling is pivotal in PCa progression, making it a key target for therapeutic interventions [51]. One challenge in curcumin-based therapies is its limited bioavailability, which can be addressed using nanoparticle-based delivery systems [48]. Beyond its anticancer properties, curcumin exhibits diverse pharmacological effects, including anti-inflammatory, antimicrobial, antidiabetic, antioxidant, and neuroprotective activities [78].

6.3 Breast cancer

Curcumin exerts strong anticancer effects in breast cancer by modulating critical molecular signaling pathways. It induces apoptosis and inhibits tumor growth and

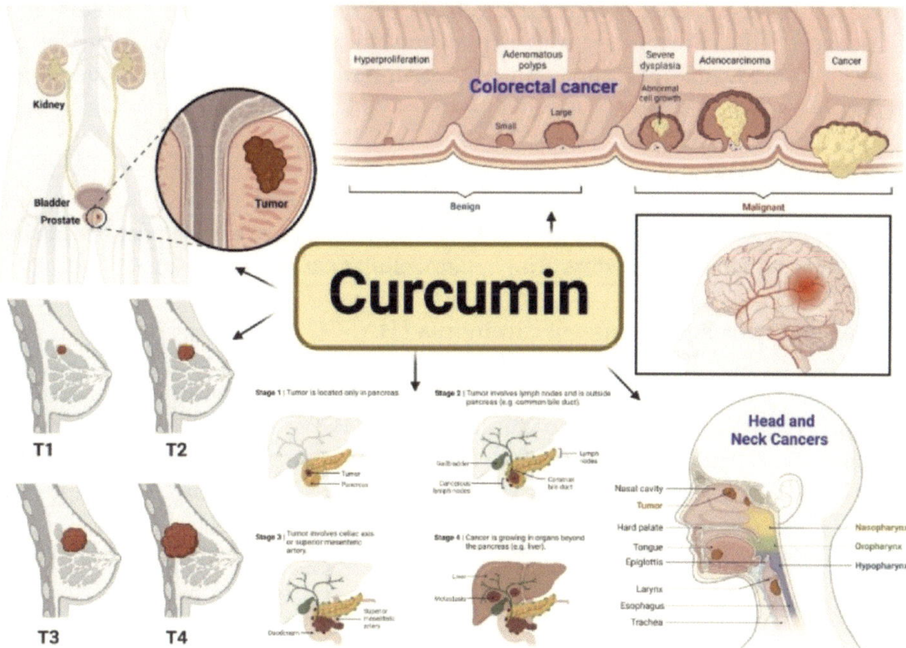

Figure 6.
Curcumin's application in the prevention and management of malignancies, including colorectal, pancreatic, breast, prostate, and head and neck cancers. https://ars.els-cdn.com/content/image/1-s2.0-S0753332223018322-gr3.jpg.

metastasis [79]. Additionally, curcumin suppresses the activity of the AP-1 transcription factor, which is associated with anti-apoptotic proteins [48]. By targeting the IL-6/STAT3 pathway, curcumin further disrupts oncogenic signaling [80]. These multifaceted actions highlight curcumin's potential both as a standalone treatment and in combination with other therapies for multiple cancers, including breast, pancreatic, prostate, oral, lung, and colorectal malignancies [76].

6.4 Colorectal cancer

Colorectal cancer (CRC) arises from a combination of genetic, environmental, and inflammatory factors [81, 82]. Curcumin's influence on gut microbiota has been explored in CRC models, where it, alongside tocotrienol-rich fractions, has been shown to alter microbial diversity, suggesting a potential therapeutic synergy in inhibiting cancer cell proliferation [83]. Dietary modifications incorporating curcumin may serve as a preventive approach against CRC development.

Curcumin has been studied extensively for its anticancer properties in various malignancies, including leukemia, liver, stomach, and prostate cancers. When combined with resveratrol, curcumin demonstrates enhanced anticancer activity, inducing apoptosis through multiple pro-apoptotic genes and signaling pathways. Studies on colorectal cell lines (DLD-1 and CaCo-2) indicate that the effectiveness of curcumin-resveratrol combinations varies based on dosage, with IC50 values of 66.21 and 71.8 μM, respectively [84].

Curcumin also induces cell cycle arrest at the G1 and G2/M phases, suppressing tumor growth through interactions with molecular targets. Animal models have provided further evidence of curcumin's chemopreventive effects in hereditary and inflammatory CRC. Formulations incorporating curcumin into nanoparticles have improved its bioavailability, enhancing its anti-inflammatory and anticancer properties [85].

6.5 Pancreatic cancer

Curcumin-loaded emulsome nanoparticles (CurEm) have shown promise in the treatment of pancreatic, prostate, and hepatocellular carcinomas [86].

6.6 Head and neck squamous cell carcinoma (HNSCC)

Head and neck cancers (HNC) are aggressive and difficult to treat, often arising from lifestyle factors or human papillomavirus (HPV) infections. Enhancing curcumin's therapeutic efficacy through novel formulations or combination therapies may provide new treatment options for HNC, potentially leading to clinical applications [87].

7. Curcumin's influence on cancer cell growth and proliferation

7.1 Induction of apoptosis and inhibition of cell proliferation

Curcumin's anticancer effects are largely mediated by its ability to induce apoptosis and suppress cell proliferation [88]. It disrupts the cell cycle, thereby inhibiting cancer cell growth [89, 90]. Studies have evaluated dietary compounds for their impact on cell viability, genotoxicity, and apoptotic pathways in human cancer cell lines [91].

Research has also demonstrated that curcumin increases the sensitivity of *Saccharomyces cerevisiae* cells to toxic effects, supporting its role in preventing uncontrolled cell growth [92, 93]. Experimental studies have shown that certain dietary phytochemicals suppress both cancerous and non-cancerous cell proliferation. The comet assay has been used to determine the optimal doses at which these compounds induce DNA damage, further validating their anticancer effects [94, 95].

In a study on cadmium chloride exposure, its impact on lung cancer (A549), hepatocellular carcinoma (HepG2), and normal lung cells (Wi38) was assessed, demonstrating the increased vulnerability of cancer cells [96]. The expression levels of apoptotic genes such as p53, Bax, and Bcl-2 were measured using real-time polymerase chain reaction (PCR). Results indicated that gold nanorods (AuNRs) influenced apoptosis-related gene expression, significantly downregulating Bcl-2 while upregulating p53 and Bax. This shift in apoptotic regulators facilitates the release of cytochrome c from mitochondria, triggering caspase activation and programmed cell death (**Figure 7**) [97].

7.2 Numerous studies

Various studies have demonstrated that curcumin exhibits anticancer properties through multiple mechanism. Findings suggest that curcumin exhibits limited bioavailability, likely due to poor absorption [97]. A pilot study examining standardized curcumin extracts in colorectal cancer patients indicated that curcumin's

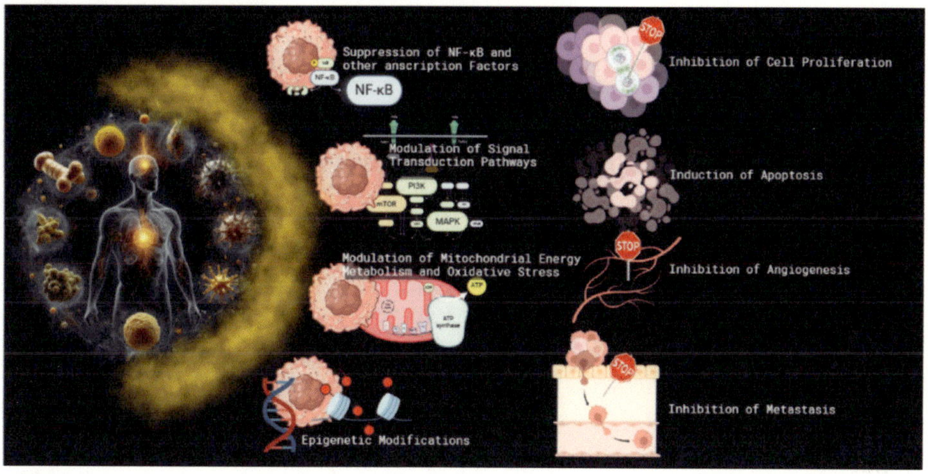

Figure 7.
Mechanisms of curcumin in cancer prevention. Curcumin, a polyphenolic compound found in turmeric, employs multiple mechanisms to prevent cancer development. It induces apoptosis by arresting the cell cycle, inhibiting cell proliferation, and modulating apoptotic proteins. Additionally, curcumin disrupts key signal transduction pathways such as PI3K/Akt/mTOR and MAPK/ERK while suppressing crucial transcription factors like NF-κB, STAT3, and AP-1. Curcumin also plays a role in inhibiting angiogenesis and metastasis by downregulating vascular endothelial growth factor (VEGF), VEGF receptor 2 (VEGFR2), and matrix metalloproteinases (MMPs). It is anticancer "Curcumin exhibits potent anticancer properties by targeting multiple cellular mechanisms, including apoptosis, signal transduction pathways, angiogenesis, and metastasis inhibition." https://www.mdpi.com/cancers/cancers-16-02580/article_deploy/html/images/cancers-16-02580-g003.png.

bioavailability in humans might also be restricted [98]. Research conducted *in vitro* using human and rat hepatocyte preparations, as well as in vivo studies in rats and mice, has provided insights into curcumin metabolism [99].

A recent meta-analysis demonstrated that curcumin enhances antioxidant levels in individuals susceptible to oxidative stress (OS) [100]. This effect is attributed to its ability to scavenge free radicals and inhibit malondialdehyde production [101]. The extent to which curcumin reduces OS depends on both the dosage and duration of treatment [102].

After oral ingestion, only a small fraction of curcumin is absorbed and metabolized, while the majority is excreted unchanged in feces [103]. Curcumin metabolism occurs in two distinct phases. During the first phase, enterocytes and hepatocytes facilitate reduction reactions involving enzymes such as alcohol dehydrogenase, nicotinamide adenine dinucleotide phosphate (NADPH)-dependent reductase, and an unidentified microsomal enzyme [97]. These enzymatic processes produce reduced metabolites, including dihydrocurcumin, tetrahydrocurcumin, hexahydrocurcumin, and octahydrocurcumin (also known as hexahydrocurcuminol) [98].

In both *in vitro* and *in vivo* settings, curcumin and its reduced metabolites undergo conjugation with glucuronic acid and sulfate. The glucuronidation and sulfation processes are catalyzed by glucuronyl transferase and sulfotransferase, respectively, and occur in both the liver and intestines of humans and rats [99].

Consuming curcumin in its natural form, such as fresh or powdered turmeric, rather than as a supplement, enhances bioavailability [100]. This improvement may result from the influence of the turmeric matrix or interactions between curcumin and other turmeric constituents [101]. Additionally, utilizing nanoformulations has been explored as a strategy to increase curcumin's bioavailability

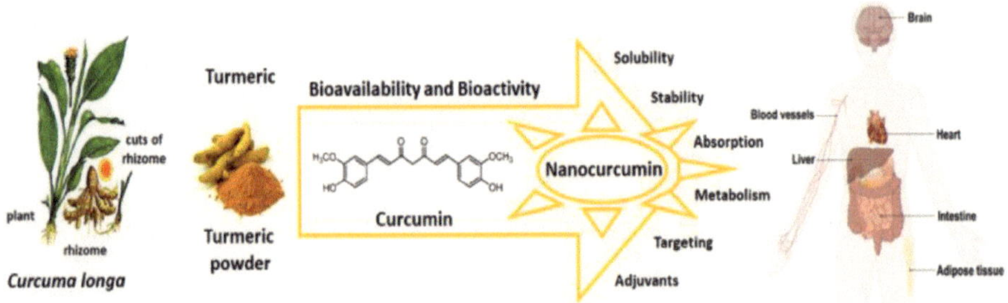

Figure 8.
Techniques for curcumin nanoformulation enhance solubility, stability, absorption, and targeted delivery while also improving bioavailability and bioactivity [104].

and bioactivity [102]. Enhancing curcumin levels through these advanced formulations may improve its therapeutic potential, particularly due to its potent antioxidant properties **Figure 8** [103].

7.3 Curcumin formulations for enhanced bioavailability

A comprehensive review of clinical trials has examined multiple generations of curcumin formulations, assessing their efficacy and safety across various diseases. This includes an overview of the formulations' dosage, duration, and mechanisms of action. Additionally, their advantages and limitations have been critically analyzed in comparison to placebos and standard treatments. The integrative approach in next-generation formulations aims to overcome bioavailability and safety challenges while

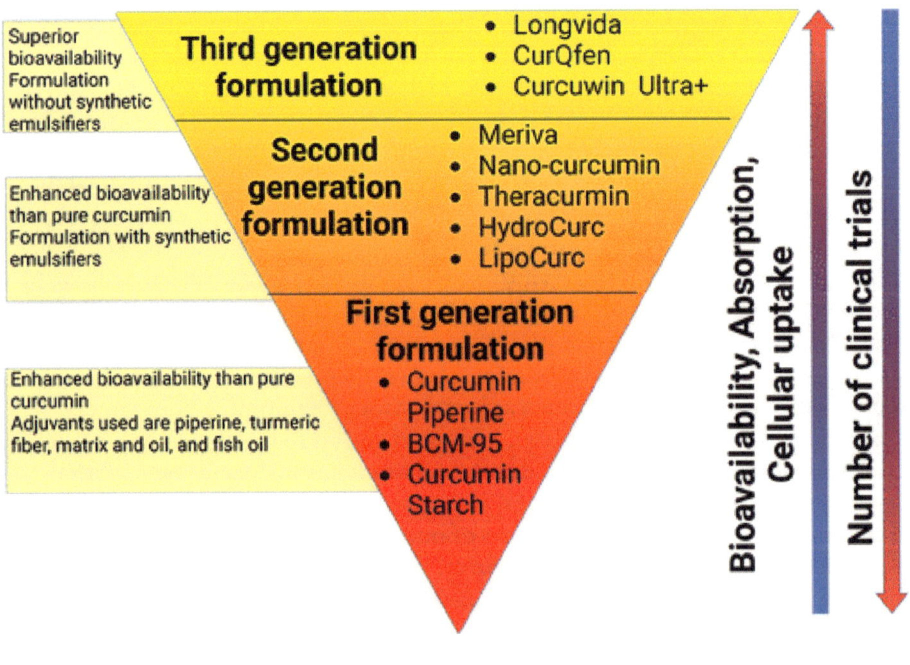

Figure 9.
Formulations of curcumin for increased bioavailability.

minimizing adverse effects. These advancements may also contribute to the prevention and treatment of complex chronic diseases (See **Figure 9** [105]).

8. Mechanisms and activities of curcumin

Curcumin has shown potential as a more effective treatment compared to existing therapies. However, its low bioavailability remains a major challenge for its use as a therapeutic agent. If this issue is addressed, curcumin-based drugs for Alzheimer's disease (AD) could become a viable option [106]. Additionally, curcumin plays a significant role in human health (**Figure 10**).

Analysis of the pathogenic pathways caused by arecoline and the mechanism of action of curcumin in the prevention and treatment of oral submucous fibrosis **Figure 11** [107].

8.1 Categories of curcumin-related products

Curcumin-related substances can be classified into five main categories:

Turmeric (T): Derived from raw *Curcuma longa* rhizomes.

Turmeric Extract (TE): Obtained by solvent extraction of fresh or dried *C. longa* rhizomes.

Curcuminoid-Enriched Turmeric Extract (CTE): A concentrated solvent extract that forms a deep yellow precipitate at lower temperatures.

Curcuminoid-Enriched Material (CEM): Further purified from CTE using large-scale chromatographic techniques.

Curcumin (CUR): A single, highly purified chemical compound, often used as a metrological or reference material.

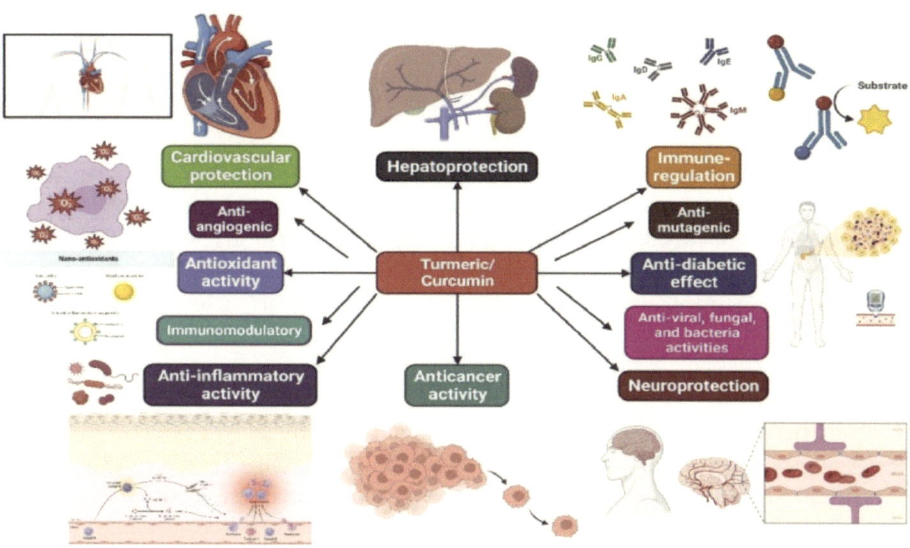

Figure 10.
Curcumin's effects on human health, including cancer. Curcumin may help control diabetes, alleviate arthritis, and lessen inflammation in bowel disorders because of its anticancer, anti-inflammatory, antioxidant, and neuroprotective qualities. https://ars.els-cdn.com/content/image/1-s2.0-S0753332223018322-gr2.jpg.

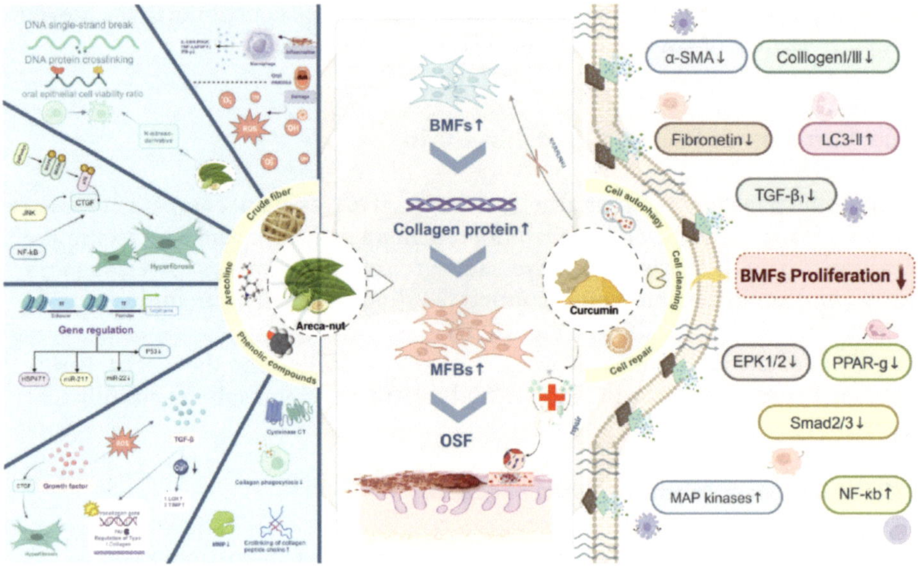

Figure 11.
Oral submucous fibrosis mechanisms and mechanisms of action. Mechanism of curcumin in the prevention and treatment of oral submucosal fibrosis and progress in clinical application research.

It is important to distinguish between curcumin as a pure compound and the various preparations often referred to by the same name. The lack of precise chemical characterization among crude turmeric (T), extracts (TE), enriched materials (CTE, CEM), and even highly purified curcumin complicates the interpretation of biological data. This ambiguity raises concerns about the validity of results obtained from different preparations, as their composition may vary significantly [108]. Furthermore, attributing the biological activity of complex mixtures solely to curcumin can be challenging, regardless of its prominence [109].

8.2 Antiviral properties

Curcumin, the primary curcuminoid in turmeric, exhibits broad-spectrum antimicrobial properties, including antibacterial, antiviral, and antifungal activity [110]. Studies suggest that curcuminoid Me23 may help mitigate the effects of COVID-19, particularly when the central nervous system is involved [111]. Additionally, curcumin has demonstrated antiviral capabilities against various viruses, as summarized in **Table 3** [112].

9. Hepatoprotective effects

Curcumin has been shown to restore oxidative balance by reversing changes in malondialdehyde (MDA) levels, catalase activity, and key antioxidant enzymes such as superoxide dismutase (SOD) and glutathione (GSH). Additionally, it helps regulate electrolyte balance, reduces liver fibrosis, and lowers biomarkers associated

Pathway/process	Antiviral activity	Virus
Actin filament organization	Viral entry	Dengue virus Viral hemorrhagic septicemia virus
	Replication	Dengue virus
Anti-inflammation	Replication	Human immunodeficiency virus
Antioxidation	Replication	Human immunodeficiency virus
APE1 redox reactions	Replication	Kaposi's sarcoma-associated herpesvirus
Cell lipogenesis	Replication	Dengue virus
Cleavage of eIF4G	Protein expression	Enterovirus 71
Conformation of viral/cellular surface proteins	Viral attachment	Zika virus Chikungunya virus Vesicular stomatitis virus
		Human respiratory syncytial virus
HSC71 expression	Viral entry	Viral hemorrhagic septicemia virus
NF-κB signaling	Replication	Influenza A virus
	Viral egress	Herpes simplex virus 2
PKCδ phosphorylation	Protein expression?	Enterovirus 71
ROS production	Viricidal	Norovirus
Lipid raft formation		Bovine herpes virus 1
Viral enzymes	Viral egress Viral protease	Influenza A virus Dengue virus
Viral proteins	Viral entry	Influenza A virus Porcine reproductive and respiratory syndrome virus
	Viral protein degradation	Human immunodeficiency virus
	Viricidal	Norovirus

Table 3.
Pathways and mechanisms influenced by curcumin and its analogs.

with liver damage. These findings suggest that curcumin may play a protective role against liver cirrhosis [113].

9.1 Antithrombotic properties

Thrombosis primarily results from platelet activation and aggregation, leading to vascular blockages that cause conditions such as heart attacks, angina, and ischemic stroke. Given the increasing prevalence of thrombotic diseases, there is a growing need for safer and more effective treatments. Curcumin has demonstrated antithrombotic properties by inhibiting platelet activity, thereby aiding in the prevention and treatment of cardiovascular diseases (CVDs). It has also been found to help clear circulatory blockages. When taken orally, curcumin is considered a safe alternative with no reported adverse effects. Studies

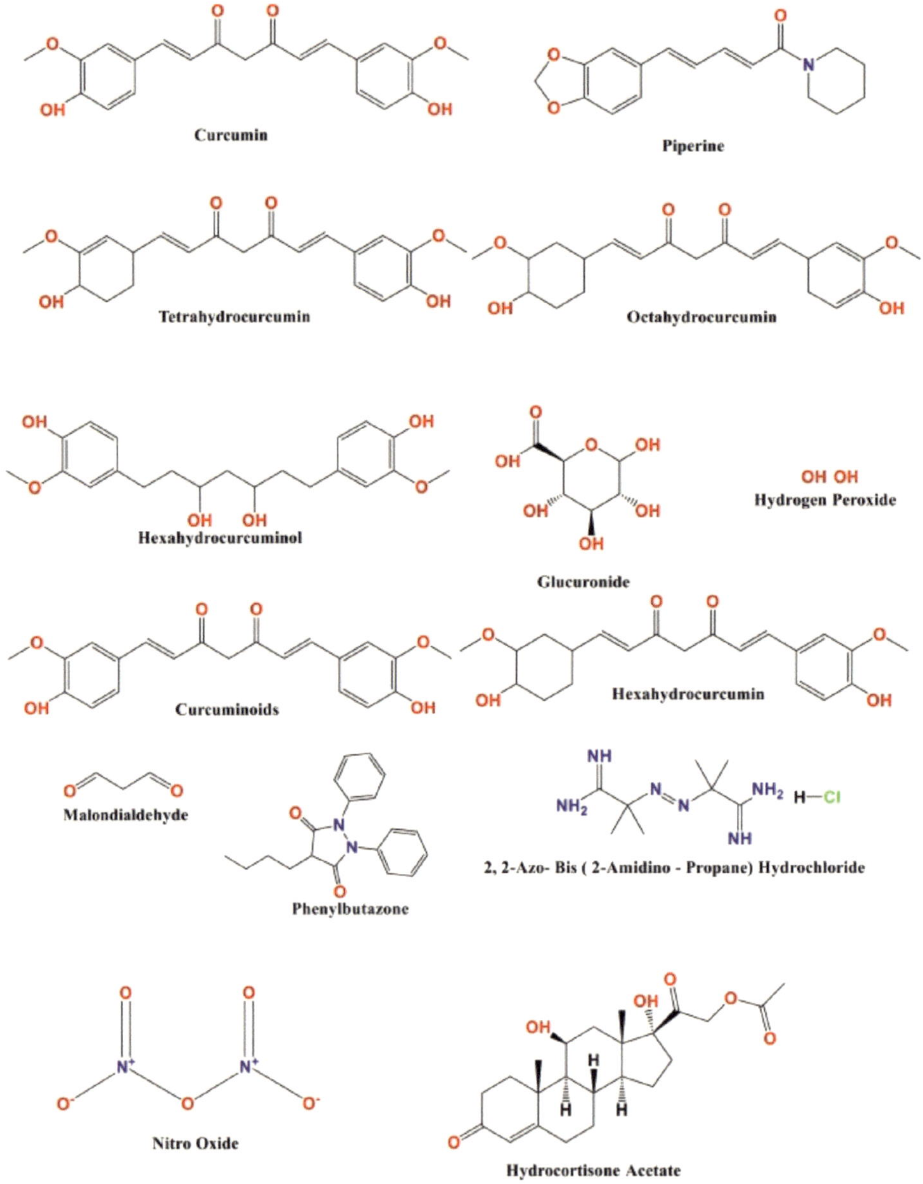

Figure 12.
Both human health and illnesses can benefit from these chemicals. https://ars.els-cdn.com/content/image/1-s2.0-S0753332223018322-gr4.jpg.

indicate that curcumin can reduce platelet aggregation induced by platelet-activating factor (PAF) *in vitro*, further supporting its potential as an antithrombotic agent [114].

9.2 Potential side effects of curcumin

While curcumin has shown promise in treating various conditions, including cancer, high concentrations may have cytotoxic effects. Excessive curcumin exposure has been linked to the destruction of healthy cells, potentially increasing cancer risk. Research suggests that both healthy human dermal fibroblasts (HDF) and breast cancer cells (MCF7) can be affected by curcumin [115]. Additionally, significant cytotoxicity has been observed in fibroblast cell cultures following topical application [116]. The broader impact of curcumin and related compounds on human health and disease is illustrated in **Figure 12**.

10. Medicinal benefits

Curcumin continues to attract attention in medicine, particularly for its potential in combating infections and cancer. Its strong antioxidant and anti-inflammatory properties make it a promising candidate for managing inflammatory bowel diseases, diabetes, and cardiovascular disorders (**Figure 13**).

The biological effects of curcumin stem from its ability to regulate specific enzymes and cellular pathways [117]. This contributes to its anticancer properties, as it can induce apoptosis and inhibit tumor growth. Studies have shown that curcumin is effective against various cancers, including brain tumors, squamous cell carcinoma of the head and neck, as well as breast, lung, kidney, uterine, cervical, and prostate cancers. Additionally, curcumin has demonstrated the ability to reduce chemoresistance in multiple malignancies. By mimicking estrogen, curcumin and its derivatives compete for cellular entry *via* aryl hydrocarbon receptors. Breast cancer cell lines such as BT-549, BT-20, MDA-MB-468, MDA-MB-231, and MCF-7 have been used to study the potential benefits of co-delivering curcuminoid derivatives. The therapeutic effects of curcumin and its derivatives are linked to multiple mechanisms, including the generation of reactive oxygen species (ROS), modulation of protein kinase activity, regulation of pro-apoptotic factors, inhibition of histone deacetylase

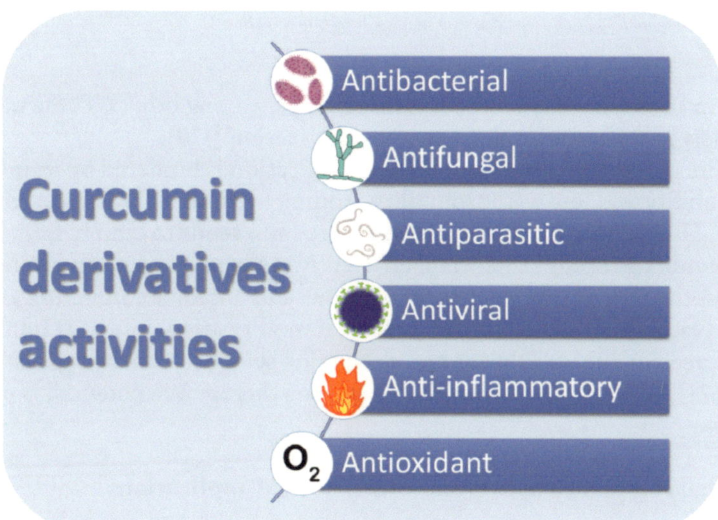

Figure 13.
Derivatives of curcumin and their biological activity.

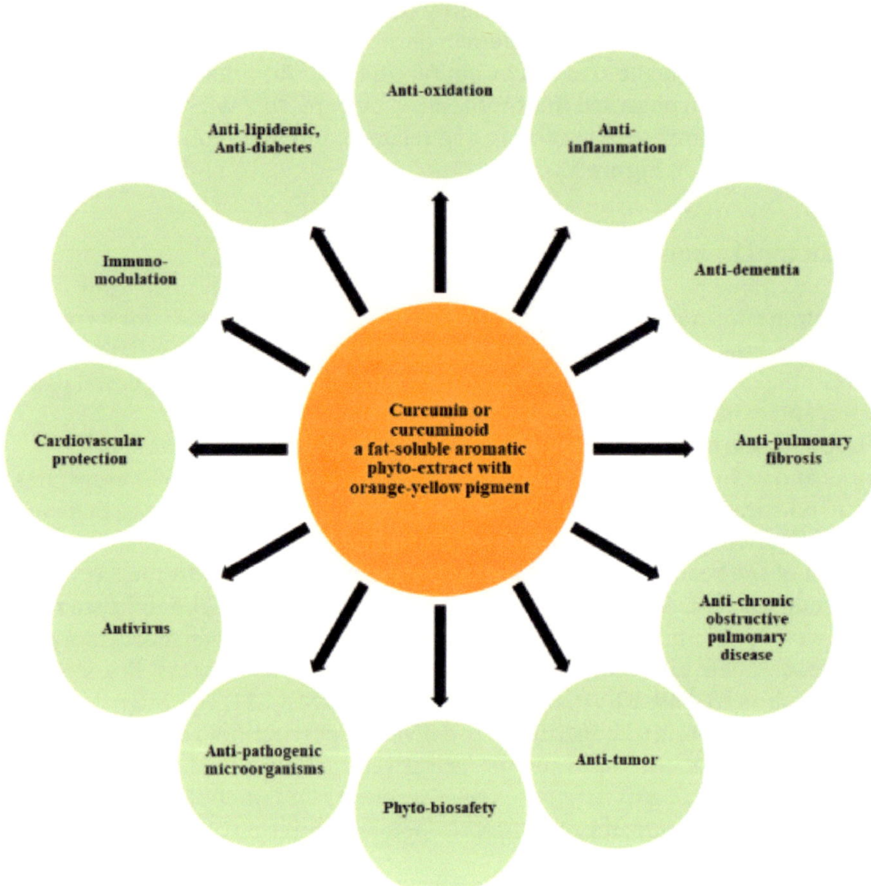
Anti-oxidation
Anti-inflammation
Anti-dementia
Anti-pulmonary fibrosis
Anti-chronic obstructive pulmonary disease
Anti-tumor
Phyto-biosafety
Anti-pathogenic microorganisms
Antivirus
Cardiovascular protection
Immuno-modulation
Anti-lipidemic, Anti-diabetes
Curcumin or curcuminoid a fat-soluble aromatic phyto-extract with orange-yellow pigment

Figure 14.
Curcuminoids have a variety of therapeutic uses. Alpha-amylase in saliva.

and telomerase, and interaction with efflux pumps, among others. These mechanisms form the basis of curcumin's role in chemosensitization [118].

Despite its potential, curcumin's clinical application is hindered by its poor chemical stability and low water solubility, leading to limited absorption when taken orally [119]. Due to its hydrophobic nature, curcumin tends to bind to fatty acyl chains in membrane lipids rather than efficiently entering the cytoplasm, restricting its cellular uptake. To overcome these limitations and enhance curcumin's anticancer properties, researchers are exploring structural modifications aimed at improving stability, increasing bioavailability, and enhancing selective toxicity against cancer cells [120, 121]. A detailed overview of curcumin's therapeutic potential is presented in **Figure 14**.

10.1 Chemical composition, origins, and historical applications

Curcumin, the primary curcuminoid in turmeric (*Curcuma longa*) from the Zingiberaceae family, possesses a unique chemical structure:

1,7-bis(4-hydroxy-3-methoxyphenyl)-1,6-heptadiene-3,5-dione. This structure enables keto-enol tautomerism, which varies depending on environmental pH and influences curcumin's chemical stability and therapeutic effects. This characteristic plays a crucial role in curcumin's biological interactions, particularly its anti-inflammatory and antioxidant functions [122].

Historically, turmeric has been used as both a spice and a dye. The extraction of curcumin in the early nineteenth century marked a transition toward its medical significance. Traditional medicine systems have employed curcumin for centuries to address ailments such as wounds, infections, and digestive disorders [123]. Modern research supports its anti-inflammatory, free-radical scavenging, and anticancer properties, validated by extensive *in vivo* and *in vitro* studies [124].

11. Therapeutic benefits of curcumin and nano-curcumin in age-related diseases

11.1 Neurological disorders

Astrocytes, the most prevalent glial cells in the central nervous system, play a significant role in neurological disorders and brain injuries. Research suggests curcumin may aid in mitigating brain aging and neurodegenerative diseases due to its antioxidant, anti-inflammatory, and free-radical scavenging properties [125].

Curcumin has shown promise in enhancing cognitive and motor functions in middle-aged and older adults. It has also been linked to increased expression of the CISD2 gene, which declines with age and contributes to neurodegeneration. Studies on animal models of Alzheimer's disease indicate that curcumin reduces oxidative stress and inflammation, leading to improved neurological health [104]. Although some trials reported adverse effects, overall findings suggest curcumin may help modulate inflammation and improve clinical outcomes in neurodegenerative disorders [126].

11.2 Atherosclerosis

Curcumin, a polyphenolic compound found in *C. longa* rhizomes, exhibits anti-inflammatory, antioxidant, and anti-atherosclerotic effects. Atherosclerosis involves the thickening and hardening of arteries, impairing blood flow and increasing the risk of strokes and heart attacks [127].

Curcumin-based treatments influence key signaling pathways related to inflammation, gene transcription, and cholesterol regulation. These mechanisms contribute to preventing atherosclerosis and highlight curcumin's potential therapeutic value in cardiovascular diseases [128].

11.3 Reproductive system disorders

Curcumin's anti-inflammatory, anti-apoptotic, and antioxidant properties benefit ovarian health. Aging leads to apoptosis-driven depletion of ovarian follicles, but curcumin supplementation has been shown to increase follicle count, ovarian volume, and hormone levels, including estrogen and anti-Müllerian hormone [129].

Additionally, curcumin enhances embryo development and egg maturation, while reducing oxidative stress. Its antimicrobial, antiproliferative, and antiangiogenic effects have been linked to the suppression of key cancer-related pathways, making it a promising candidate for ovarian cancer treatment [130].

11.4 Skeletal muscle health

Curcumin helps combat skeletal muscle aging by neutralizing reactive oxygen species (ROS) and enhancing antioxidant enzyme activity. Studies in older rats indicate that curcumin supplementation improves muscle mass and function, particularly by increasing plantar muscle strength. Additionally, curcumin has demonstrated protective effects against skeletal muscle ischemia-reperfusion injury [131].

12. Overall health benefits

Decades of pharmacological research have demonstrated curcumin's broad-spectrum therapeutic potential. Its multitarget and multichannel properties contribute to its effectiveness in treating Alzheimer's disease, regulating blood lipid and glucose levels, and providing anticoagulant, antiplatelet, and antiviral benefits [132].

Recent findings suggest curcumin may inhibit the replication of emerging viruses, including the coronavirus. However, its poor water solubility and bioavailability remain significant challenges. Advances in curcumin formulations, including novel complexes,

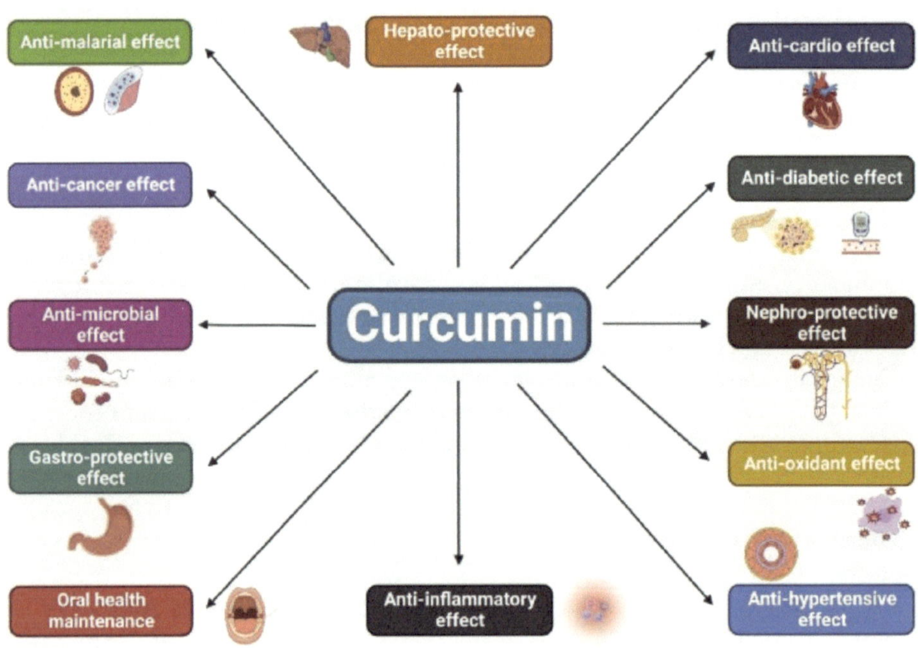

Figure 15.
Numerous studies have demonstrated that curcumin is safe, well-tolerated, and effective in the prevention and treatment of a wide range of chronic illnesses, including infectious diseases, cancer, heart disease, diabetes, neurological disorders, skin ailments, and liver problems [48]. https://ars.els-cdn.com/content/image/1-s2.0-S0753332223018322-gr5.jpg.

have aimed to overcome these limitations, improving its pharmacological efficacy. Despite these advancements, further investigation is needed to ensure the safety of curcumin-based additives and colorants, as excessive use may pose health risks [133].

By optimizing curcumin's bioavailability and safety profile, its full therapeutic potential could be harnessed for a variety of human health applications **Figure 15** [134].

13. Conclusion

Curcumin exhibits multiple therapeutic effects, influencing cellular biochemistry, physiological regulation, immunomodulation, and infection suppression, making it a valuable pharmaceutical agent. It holds potential in preventing and treating cardiovascular diseases, respiratory conditions, cancer, neurodegeneration, infections, and inflammatory disorders. Recent advancements in molecular simulation and structural studies have provided insights into its molecular interactions, though further clinical trials are necessary to confirm its efficacy in new disease treatments and infectious disease prevention.

Curcumin exerts its effects by interacting with various biochemical pathways and cellular targets. It plays a role in epigenetic regulation by modifying DNA methylation, histone structures, and microRNA expression, thereby influencing gene expression and multiple biological processes. Studies have demonstrated its ability to mitigate diabetic nephropathy by inhibiting the NLRP3 inflammasome pathway and promoting autophagy, which helps protect renal tubular epithelial cells from advanced glycation end products.

Additionally, curcumin has been found to modulate microRNA activity, such as inhibiting miR-133b to restore kidney function and miR-138 to promote wound healing. Its role in repressing miR-152-3p has been linked to accelerated wound healing in diabetic foot ulcers by reducing apoptosis and enhancing fibroblast migration and proliferation [6].

Research into the application of C3-Diagard™ Cream for treating diabetic foot ulcers has shown promising results regarding curcumin's safety and efficacy. Moreover, studies suggest that even at low concentrations, curcumin promotes the growth of placental trophoblast cells by positively influencing angiogenesis and gene expression. Further research is needed to determine whether curcumin can serve as a modulator of placental angiogenesis to support fetal development in compromised pregnancies.

In both *in vitro* and *in vivo* studies, curcumin therapy has demonstrated inhibitory effects on head and neck squamous cell carcinoma (HNSCC). This review highlights the mechanisms of action, biological activity, potential therapeutic applications, and clinical considerations of curcumin, providing valuable insights into its role in diagnosing and treating oral submucosal fibrosis and other conditions.

Acknowledgements

Our sincere gratitude is extended to the National Research Center, Egypt.

Funding

This study received no internal or external funding.

Conflict of interest

The author has no competing interests to declare.

Data availability

All data generated or analyzed during this study are included in this published article.

Consent for publication

We certify that the manuscript you have received has not been published elsewhere or is under consideration by any other journals.

Author details

Shimaa E. Rashad
Microbial Genetics Department, Biotechnology Research Institute, National Research Centre, Egypt

*Address all correspondence to: se.rashad@nrc.sci.eg; shimaar30@yahoo.com

References

[1] Hsu KY, Ho CT, Pan MH. The therapeutic potential of curcumin and its related substances in turmeric: From raw material selection to application strategies. Journal of Food and Drug Analysis. 2023;**31**(2):194-211

[2] Amalraj A, Pius A, Gopi S, Gopi S. Biological activities of Curcuminoids, other biomolecules from turmeric and their derivatives–A review. Journal of Traditional and Complementary Medicine. 2017;7:205-233

[3] JECFA. Sixty-First Report of the Joint FAO/WHO Expert Committee on Food Additives. Joint FAO/WHO Expert Committee on Food Additives (JECFA); 2004

[4] Aggarwal BB, Harikumar KB. Potential therapeutic effects of curcumin, the anti-inflammatory agent, against neurodegenerative, cardiovascular, pulmonary, metabolic, autoimmune and neoplastic diseases. The International Journal of Biochemistry & Cell Biology. 2009;**41**:40-59

[5] López-Lázaro M. Anticancer and carcinogenic properties of curcumin: Considerations for its clinical development as a cancer chemopreventive and chemotherapeutic agent. Molecular Nutrition & Food Research. 2008;**52**:S103-S127

[6] Amaroli A, Panfoli I, Bozzo M, Ferrando S, Candiani S, Ravera S. The bright side of curcumin: A narrative review of its therapeutic potential in Cancer management. Cancers. 2024;**16**(14):2580

[7] Sharifi-Rad J, Rayess YE, Rizk AA, Sadaka C, Zgheib R, Zam W, et al. Turmeric and its major compound curcumin on health: Bioactive effects and safety profiles for food, pharmaceutical, biotechnological and medicinal applications. Frontiers in Pharmacology. 2020;**11**:1021

[8] Urošević M, Nikolić L, Gajić I, Nikolić V, Dinić A, Miljković V. Curcumin: Biological activities and modern pharmaceutical forms. Antibiotics. 2022;**11**:135

[9] Ramirez-Ahumada MDC, Timmermann BN, Gang DR. Biosynthesis of curcuminoids and gingerols in turmeric (*Curcuma longa*) and ginger (*Zingiber Officinale*): Identification of curcuminoid synthase and hydroxycinnamoyl-coa thioesterases. Phytochemistry. 2006;**67**:2017-2029

[10] Kriplani P, Guarve K. Physicochemical and biological aspects of curcumin: A review. Natural Products Journal. 2020;**11**:318-343

[11] Matthewman C, Krishnakumar IM, Swick AG. Review: Bioavailability and efficacy of "free" curcuminoids from curcumagalactomannoside (CGM) curcumin formulation. Nutrition Research Reviews. 2024;**37**:14-31

[12] Stati G, Rossi F, Sancilio S, Basile M, Di Pietro R. *Curcuma longa* hepatotoxicity: A baseless accusation. Cases assessed for causality using RUCAM method. Frontiers in Pharmacology. 2021;**12**:780330

[13] Giacomo Di S, Briz O, Vitalone A, Di Sotto A. Editorial: Natural products and hepatic health: Light and shadows. Frontiers in Pharmacology. 2022;**13**:868207

[14] Hussain Y, Abdullah, Khan F, Alsharif KF, Alzahrani KJ, Saso L,

et al. Regulatory effects of curcumin on platelets: An update and future directions. Biomedicine. 2022;**10**:3180

[15] Olas B. The antioxidant, anti-platelet and anti-coagulant properties of phenolic compounds, associated with modulation of hemostasis and cardiovascular disease, and their possible effect on COVID-19. Nutrients. 2022;**14**:1390

[16] Mashayekhi-Sardoo H, Mashayekhi-Sardoo A, Roufogalis BD, Jamialahmadi T, Sahebkar A. Impact of curcumin on microsomal enzyme activities: Drug interaction and chemopreventive studies. Current Medicinal Chemistry. 2021;**28**:7122-7140

[17] Li R, Xiang C, Ye M, Li H-F, Zhang X, Guo D-A. Qualitative and quantitative analysis of Curcuminoids in herbal medicines derived from *Curcuma* species. Food Chemistry. 2011;**126**:1890-1895

[18] Wu H, Liu Z, Zhang Y, Gao B, Li Y, He X, et al. Chemical composition of turmeric (*Curcuma longa* L.) ethanol extract and its antimicrobial activities and free radical scavenging capacities. Food. 2024;**13**(10):1550. DOI: 10.3390/Foods13101550

[19] Poudel A, Pandey J, Lee H-K. Geographical discrimination in Curcuminoids content of turmeric assessed by rapid UPLC-DAD validated analytical method. Molecules. 2019;**24**:1805

[20] Mohaw T. Taiwan Herbal Pharmacopeia (IV). Ministry of Health and Welfare (MOHW); 2021

[21] Commission CP. Pharmacopoeia of People's Republic of China. Beijing: China Medical Science Press; 2020. p. 138

[22] Jiang T, Ghosh R, Charcosset C. Extraction, purification and applications of curcumin from plant materials-A comprehensive review. Trends in Food Science and Technology. 2021;**112**:419-430

[23] Zhu J, Sanidad KZ, Sukamtoh E, Zhang G. Potential roles of chemical degradation in the biological activities of curcumin. Food & Function. 2017;**8**:907-914

[24] Zielinska H, Alves V, Marques A, Durazzo M, Lucarini TF, Alves M, et al. Souto properties, extraction methods, and delivery systems for curcumin as a natural source of beneficial health effects. Medicina. 2020;**56**(7):336

[25] Kanubaddi KR, Yang SH, Wu LW, Lee CH, Weng CF. Nanoparticle-conjugated nutraceuticals exert prospectively palliative of amyloid aggregation. International Journal of Nanomedicine. 2018;**13**:8473-8485

[26] Roxo DF, Arcaro CA, Gutierres VO, Costa MC, Oliveira JO, Lima TFO, et al. Curcumin combined with metformin decreases glycemia and dyslipidemia, and increases paraoxonase activity in diabetic rats. Diabetology and Metabolic Syndrome. 2019;**11**:33

[27] Ahmad RS, Hussain MB, Sultan MT, Arshad MS, Waheed M, Shariati MA, et al. Biochemistry, safety, pharmacological activities, and clinical applications of turmeric: A mechanistic review. Evidence-based Complementary and Alternative Medicine : eCAM. 2020;**2020**(1):1-14:7656919. DOI: 10.1155/2020/7656919

[28] Gopi S, Thomas S, Kunnumakkara AB, Aggarwal BB, Aggarwal A. Evaluation and clinical comparison studies on liposomal and non-liposomal ascorbic acid (vitamin C) and their enhanced bioavailability. Journal of Liposome

Research. 2020;**31**(4):356-364. DOI: 10.1080/08982104.2020.1820521

[29] Asbaghi O, Ashtary-Larky D, Bagheri R, Nazarian B, Pourmirzaei Olyaei H, Rezaei Kelishadi M, et al. Beneficial effects of folic acid supplementation on lipid markers in adults: A GRADE-assessed systematic review and dose-response meta-analysis of data from 21,787 participants in 34 randomized controlled trials. Critical Reviews in Food Science and Nutrition. 2021;**62**(30):8435-8453. DOI: 10.1080/10408398.2021.1928598

[30] Kocaadam B, Şanlier N. Curcumin, an active component of turmeric (*Curcuma longa*), and its effects on health. Critical Reviews in Food Science and Nutrition. 2017;**57**:2889-2895

[31] Mansouri K, Rasoulpoor S, Daneshkhah A, Abolfathi S, Salari N, Mohammadi M, et al. Clinical effects of curcumin in enhancing cancer therapy: A systematic review. BMC Cancer. 2020;**20**:791

[32] Tabrizi R, Vakili S, Akbari M, Mirhosseini N, Lankarani KB, Rahimi M, et al. The effects of curcumin-containing supplements on biomarkers of inflammation and oxidative stress: A systematic review and meta-analysis of randomized controlled trials. Phytotherapy Research. 2019;**33**:253-262

[33] Tavakol S, Zare S, Hoveizi E, Tavakol B, Rezayat SM. The impact of the particle size of curcumin nanocarriers and the ethanol on beta_1-integrin overexpression in fibroblasts: A regenerative pharmaceutical approach in skin repair and anti-aging formulations. Daru. 2019;**27**:159-168

[34] Ardebili A, Pouriayevali MH, Aleshikh S, Zahani M, Ajorloo M, Izanloo A, et al. Antiviral therapeutic potential of curcumin: An update. Molecules. 2021;**26**(22):6994. DOI: 10.3390/Molecules26226994

[35] Mahmoudi A, Jamialahmadi T, Kesharwani P, Sahebkar A. Bioinformatic analysis of the molecular targets of curcumin in colorectal cancer. Pathology - Research and Practice. 2024;**262**:344-338

[36] Alkhathami AG, Alshahrani MY, Alshehri SA, et al. Curcumin as a potential inhibitor of Tgfβ3 computational insights for breast cancer therapy. Scientific Reports. 2025;**15**:2871. DOI: 10.1038/S41598-025-86289-0

[37] Sharma R, Mali Y, Agrawal YO, Agnihotri VV, Goyal SN. Repurposing nano curcumin: Unveiling its therapeutic potential in diabetic nephropathy. Current Drug Targets. 2025;**26**. DOI: 10.2174/0113894501326054241126043554

[38] Gokdemir GS, Gokdemir MT, Tasdemir E, et al. Importance of curcumin effect and asprosin level on glucose metabolism in diabetic rats. Medicine Science. 2023;**12**:167-174

[39] Ghasemi F, Shafiee M, Banikazemi Z, Pourhanifeh MH, Khanbabaei H, Shamshirian A, et al. Curcumin inhibits NF-kb and Wnt/B-catenin pathways in cervical cancer cells. Pathology - Research and Practice. 2019;**215**(10)

[40] Iqbal A, Ghildiyal S, Singh S, Siddiqui P, Kumari M, Arshad AM. Combinatorial effect of curcumin and tumor necrosis factor-A-related apoptosis-inducing ligand (TRAIL) in induction of apoptosis via inhibition of nuclear factor kappa activity and enhancement of caspase-3 activity in chronic myeloid cells: An: In-vitro: Study. Journal of Cancer Research and Therapeutics. 2018;**14**(Suppl. 5):S1193-S1200

[41] Das L, Vinayak M. Curcumin modulates glycolytic metabolism and inflammatory cytokines via Nrf 2 in Dalton's lymphoma ascites cells in vivo. Anti-Cancer Agents in Medicinal Chemistry. 2018;**18**(12):1779-1791

[42] Moore TL, Bowley BG, Shultz PL, Calderazzo SM, Shobin EJ, Uprety AR, et al. Oral curcumin supplementation improves fine motor function in the middle-aged rhesus monkey. Somatosensory and Motor Research. 2018;**35**(1):1-10

[43] Santos-Parker JR, Lubieniecki KL, Rossman MJ, Van HJ, Ark BCJ, Strahler TR, et al. Curcumin supplementation and motor-cognitive function in healthy middle-aged and older adults. Nutrition and Healthy Aging. 2018;**4**(4):323-333

[44] Lin C-C, Chiang T-H, Sun Y-Y, Lin M-S. Protective effects of CISD2 and influence of curcumin on CISD2 expression in aged animals and inflammatory cell model. Nutrients. 2019;**11**(3):700

[45] Shi L-Y, Zhang L, Li H, Liu T-L, Lai J-C, Wu Z-B, et al. Protective effects of curcumin on acrolein-induced neurotoxicity in HT22 mouse hippocampal cells. Pharmacological Reports. 2018;**70**:1040-1046

[46] Tomeh MA, Hadianamrei R, Zhao X. A review of curcumin and its derivatives as anticancer agents. International Journal of Molecular Sciences. 2019;**20**(5):1033

[47] Banerjee S, Singh SK, Chowdhury I, Lillard JW Jr, Singh R. Combinatorial effect of curcumin with docetaxel modulates apoptotic and cell survival molecules in prostate cancer. Frontiers in Bioscience. 2017;**9**:235

[48] Islam MR, Rauf A, Akash S, Trisha SI, Nasim AH, Akter M, et al. Targeted therapies of curcumin focus on its therapeutic benefits in cancers and human health: Molecular signaling pathway-based approaches and future perspectives. Biomedicine & Pharmacotherapy. 2024;**170**:116034. DOI: 10.1016/j.biopha.2023.116034. [Epub 2023 Dec 22]

[49] Kaur G, Bose S, Kataria T, Tyagi A, Singla K, Sharma S, et al. Curcumin as a potential phytoconstituent used for cancer treatment: An overview. The Natural Products Journal. 2024;**14**(3). DOI: 10.2174/2210315514666230816095321

[50] Chainoglou E, Hadjipavlou-Litina D. Curcumin analogues and derivatives with anti-proliferative and anti-inflammatory activity: Structural characteristics and molecular targets. Expert Opinion on Drug Discovery. 2019;**14**(8):821-842. DOI: 10.1080/17460441.2019.1614560. [Epub 2019 May 16]

[51] Balaji S, Jeyaraman N, Jeyaraman M, Ramasubramanian S, Muthu S, Santos GS, et al. Impact of curcumin on gut microbiome. World Journal of Experimental Medicine. 2025;**15**(1):100275. DOI: 10.5493/wjem.v15.i1.100275

[52] Pradhan AK, Maji S, Das SK, Emdad L, Sarkar D, Fisher PB. MDA-9/Syntenin/SDCBP: New insights into a unique multifunctional scaffold protein. Cancer and Metastasis Reviews. 2020;**39**:769-781

[53] Deepak KGK, Vempati R, Nagaraju GP, Dasari VR, Rao NSDN, Malla RR. Tumor microenvironment: Challenges and opportunities in targeting metastasis of triple negative breast cancer. Pharmacological Research. 2020;**153**:104683

[54] Luo X, Liu J, Wang H, Lu H. Metabolomics identified new biomarkers for the precise diagnosis of pancreatic cancer and associated tissue metastasis. Pharmacological Research. 2020;**156**:104805

[55] Ashrafizadeh M, Zarrabi A, Hashemipour M, Vosough M, Najafi M, Shahinozzaman M, et al. Sensing the scent of death: Modulation of micrornas by curcumin in gastrointestinal cancers. Pharmacological Research. 2020;**160**:105199

[56] Shafabakhsh R, Pourhanifeh MH, Mirzaei HR, Sahebkar A, Asemi Z, Mirzaei H. Targeting regulatory T cells by curcumin: A potential for cancer immunotherapy. Pharmacological Research. 2019;**147**:104353

[57] Zoi V, Kyritsis AP, Galani V, Lazari D, Sioka C, Voulgaris S, et al. The role of curcumin in cancer: A focus on the PI3K/Akt pathway. Cancers (Basel). 2024;**16**(8):1554. DOI: 10.3390/Cancers16081554

[58] Yip HYK, Papa A. Signaling pathways in cancer: Therapeutic targets, combinatorial treatments, and new developments. Cells. 2021;**10**:659. DOI: 10.3390/Cells10030659

[59] Ochoa-Sanchez A, Sahare P, Pathak S, Banerjee A, Estevez M, Duttaroy AK, et al. Evaluation of the synergistic effects of curcumin-resveratrol co-loaded biogenic silica on colorectal cancer cells. Frontiers in Pharmacology. 2024;**15**:1341773. DOI: 10.3389/Fphar.2024.1341773

[60] Jiang E, Chen X, Bi Y, Pan C, Li X, Lan X. Curcumin inhibits oxidative stress and apoptosis induced by H_2O_2 in bovine adipose-derived stem cells (Badscs). Animals. 2024;**14**(23):3421. DOI: 10.3390/Ani14233421

[61] Wu J, Liu J, Li Z, Dong X, Wang L. Curcumin promotes the proliferation, migration, and angiogenesis of Huvecs to improve atherosclerosis through the Wnt/B-catenin pathway. Journal of Biological Regulators and Homeostatic Agents. 2024;**38**(5):4057-4064. DOI: 10.23812/j.biol.regul.homeost.agents.20243805.321

[62] Basak S, Srinivas V, Mallepogu A, Duttaroy AK. Curcumin stimulates angiogenesis through VEGF and expression of HLA-G in first-trimester human placental trophoblasts. Cell Biology International. 2020;**44**(5):1237-1251

[63] Lee Y-H, Chen Y-Y, Yeh Y-L, Wang Y-J, Chen R-J. Stilbene compounds inhibit tumor growth by the induction of cellular senescence and the inhibition of telomerase activity. International Journal of Molecular Sciences. 2019;**20**(11):2716

[64] Barnes RP, Fouquerel E, Opresko PL. The impact of oxidative DNA damage and stress on telomere homeostasis. Mechanisms of Ageing and Development. 2019;**177**:37-45

[65] Gonzalez-Hunt CP, Wadhwa M, Sanders LH. DNA damage by oxidative stress: Measurement strategies for two genomes. Current Opinion in Toxicology. 2018;**7**:87-94

[66] Eghbaliferiz S, Farhadi F, Barreto GE, Majeed M, Sahebkar A. Effects of curcumin on neurological diseases: Focus on astrocytes. Pharmacological Reports. 2020;**72**:769-782

[67] Parikh K, Kathawala J, Li C, Chen Z, Shan X, Cao XF, et al. Garg curcumin-loaded self-nanomicellizing solid dispersion system: Part II: In vivo safety and efficacy assessment against behavior deficit in Alzheimer disease drug. Drug

Delivery and Translational Research. 2018;**8**(5):1406-1420

[68] Mohseni M, Sahebkar A, Askari G, Johnston TP, Alikiaii B, Bagherniya M. The clinical use of curcumin on neurological disorders: An updated systematic review of clinical trials. Phytotherapy Research. 2021;**35**(12):6862-6882

[69] Singh L, Sharma S, Xu S, Tewari D, Fang J. Curcumin as a natural remedy for atherosclerosis: A pharmacological review. Molecules. 2021;**26**(13):4036

[70] Kamal DAM, Salamt N, Yusuf ANM, Kashim MIAM, Mokhtar MH. Potential health benefits of curcumin on female reproductive disorders: A review. Nutrients. 2021;**13**(9):3126

[71] Azami SH, Nazarian H, Abdollahifar MA, Eini F, Farsani MA, Novin MG. The antioxidant curcumin postpones ovarian aging in young and middle-aged mice. Reproduction, Fertility, and Development. 2020;**32**(3):292-303

[72] Mohebbati R, Anaeigoudari A, Khazdair M. The effects of *Curcuma longa* and curcumin on reproductive systems. Endocrine Regulations. 2017;**51**(4):220-228

[73] Feng W, Wang H, Zhang P, Gao C, Tao J, Ge Z, et al. Modulation of gut microbiota contributes to curcumin-mediated attenuation of hepatic steatosis in rats. Biochimica et Biophysica Acta. 2017;**1861**(7):1801-1812

[74] Cani PD. Human gut microbiome: Hopes, threats and promises. Gut. 2018;**67**(9):1716-1725

[75] Adak MRK. An insight into gut microbiota and its functionalities. Cellular and Molecular Life Sciences. 2019;**76**(3):473-493

[76] Di M, F, Margarucci S, Galderisi U, Crispi S, Peluso G. Curcumin, gut microbiota, and neuroprotection. Nutrients. 2019;**11**(10):2426

[77] Servida S, Piontini A, Gori F, Tomaino L, Moroncini G, De Gennaro Colonna V, et al. Curcumin and gut microbiota: A narrative overview with focus on glycemic control. International Journal of Molecular Sciences. 2024;**25**(14):7710. DOI: 10.3390/Ijms25147710

[78] Faralli E, Shekarforoush F, Ajalloueian AC, Mendes IS. Chronakis in vitro permeability enhancement of curcumin across Caco-2 cells monolayers using electrospun xanthan-chitosan nanofibers. Carbohydrate Polymers. 2019;**206**:38-47

[79] Islam T, Koboziev I, Albracht-Schulte K, Mistretta B, Scoggin S, Yosofvand M, et al. Curcumin reduces adipose tissue inflammation and alters gut microbiota in diet-induced obese male mice. Molecular Nutrition & Food Research. 2021;**65**(22):e2100274

[80] Burge K, Gunasekaran A, Eckert J, Chaaban H. Curcumin and intestinal inflammatory diseases: Molecular mechanisms of protection. International Journal of Molecular Sciences. 2019;**20**

[81] Zhu J, He L. The modulatory effects of curcumin on the gut microbiota: A potential strategy for disease treatment and health promotion. Microorganisms. 2024;**12**

[82] Cui C, Han Y, Li H, Yu H, Zhang B, Li G. Curcumin-driven reprogramming of the gut microbiota and metabolome ameliorates motor deficits and neuroinflammation in a mouse model of Parkinson's disease. Frontiers in

Cellular and Infection Microbiology. 2022;**12**:887407

[83] Anas M, Falak A, Khan A, et al. Therapeutic potential and agricultural benefits of curcumin: A comprehensive review of health and sustainability applications. Journal of Umm Al-Qura University for Applied Sciences. 2024:1-16. DOI: 10.1007/S43994-024-00200-7

[84] Alam MS, Anwar MJ, Maity MK, Azam F, Jaremko M, Emwas A-H. The dynamic role of curcumin in mitigating human illnesses: Recent advances in therapeutic applications. Pharmaceuticals. 2024;**17**(12):1674. DOI: 10.3390/Ph17121674

[85] Roy S, Paul S, Mukherjee S, De P, Mukherjee A. Unraveling mechanism and enhancing selectivity of A Ru^{II}-bis-bipyridyl-morphocumin complex with RAFT-generated glycopolymer exploiting Warburg effect in cancer. Chemistry – A European Journal. 2024;**31**:8. DOI: 10.1002/Chem.202403695

[86] Mohamed SIA, Jantan I, Haque MA. Naturally occurring immunomodulators with antitumor activity: An insight on their mechanisms of action. International Immunopharmacology. 2017;**50**:291-304

[87] Elekofehinti OO, Taiwo FA, Akinjiyan MO, et al. The potential of *Curcuma longa* L. bioactive compounds as RSK inhibitors for the treatment of prostate cancer: in silico study. African Journal of Urology. 2025;**31**:8. DOI: 10.1186/s12301-024-00469-4

[88] Wang L, Lu B, He M, Wang Y, Wang Z, Du L. Prostate cancer incidence and mortality: Global status and temporal trends in 89 countries from 2000 to 2019. Frontiers in Public Health. 2022;**10**:811044. DOI: 10.3389/fpubh.2022.811044

[89] Vasilatis DM, Lucchesi CA, Ghosh PM. Molecular similarities and differences between canine prostate cancer and human prostate cancer variants. Biomedicine. 2023;**11**(4):1100. DOI: 10.3390/biomedicines11041100

[90] Frazzoli C, Grasso G, Husaini DC, Ajibo DN, Orish FC, Orisakwe OE. Immune system and epidemics: The role of African indigenous bioactive substances. Nutrients. 2023;**15**(2):273. DOI: 10.3390/nu15020273

[91] Imran M, Insaf A, Hasan N, et al. Exploring the remarkable chemotherapeutic potential of polyphenolic antioxidants in battling various forms of cancer. Molecules. 2023;**28**(8):3475. DOI: 10.3390/molecules28083475

[92] Sivani BM, Azzeh M, Patnaik R, Pantea Stoian A, Rizzo M, Banerjee Y. Reconnoitering the therapeutic role of curcumin in disease prevention and treatment: Lessons learnt and future directions. Metabolites. 2022;**12**:639

[93] Moon D-O. Curcumin in cancer and inflammation: An in-depth exploration of molecular interactions, therapeutic potentials, and the role in disease management. International Journal of Molecular Sciences. 2024;**25**:2911

[94] Zoi V, Galani V, Lianos GD, Voulgaris S, Kyritsis AP, Alexiou GA. The role of curcumin in cancer treatment. Biomedicine. 2021;**9**:1086

[95] Screening PDQ, Board PE. Colorectal cancer screening (PDQ®). In: PDQ Cancer Information Summaries [Internet]. Bethesda, MD, USA: National Cancer Institute (US); 2023

[96] Sharma N, Alam MS, Sharma A, Garg S, Maity MK. Colorectal cancer in young adults: Epidemiology, risk factors,

development, symptoms, traditional herbal therapy and prevention. Journal of Pharmaceutical Negative Results. 2022;**14**:1370-1382

[97] Farhana L, Sarkar S, Nangia-Makker P, Yu Y, Khosla P, Levi E, et al. Natural agents inhibit colon cancer cell proliferation and alter microbial diversity in mice. Plos One. 2020

[98] Gavrilas LI, Cruceriu D, Ionescu C, Miere D, Balacescu O. Pro-apoptotic genes as new targets for single and combinatorial treatments with resveratrol and curcumin in colorectal cancer. Food & Function. 2019;**10**(6):3717-3726

[99] Pricci M, Girardi B, Giorgio F, Losurdo G, Ierardi E, Di Leo A. Curcumin and colorectal cancer: From basic to clinical evidences. International Journal of Molecular Sciences. 2020;**21**(7):2364

[100] Demirci Z, Islek Z, Siginc HI, Sahin F, Ucisik MH, Bolat ZB. Curcumin-loaded emulsome nanoparticles induces apoptosis through P53 signaling pathway in pancreatic cancer cell line PANC-1. Toxicology In Vitro. 2025;**102**

[101] Veselá K, Kejík Z, Masařík M, Babula P, Dytrych P, Martásek P, et al. Curcumin: A potential weapon in the prevention and treatment of head and neck cancer. ACS Pharmacology & Translational Science. 2024;**7**(11):3394-3418. DOI: 10.1021/Acsptsci.4c00518

[102] Zaidi SNF, Mahboob T. Hepatoprotective role of curcumin in rat liver cirrhosis. Pakistan Journal of Pharmaceutical Sciences. 2020;**33**(4)

[103] Kim K, Park KI. A review of antiplatelet activity of traditional medicinal herbs on integrative medicine studies. Evidence-based Complementary and Alternative Medicine : eCAM. 2019;**2019**:7125162

[104] Bertoncini-Silva C, Vlad A, Ricciarelli R, Giacomo Fassini P, Suen VMM, Zingg J-M. Enhancing the bioavailability and bioactivity of curcumin for disease prevention and treatment. Antioxidants. 2024;**13**(3):331. DOI: 10.3390/Antiox13030331

[105] Cianfruglia L, Minnelli C, Laudadio E, Scirè A, Armeni T. Side effects of curcumin: Epigenetic and antiproliferative implications for normal dermal fibroblast and breast cancer cells. Antioxidants. 2019;**8**(9):382

[106] Damiani E, Brugè F, Cirilli I, Marcheggiani F, Olivieri F, Armeni T, et al. Modulation of oxidative status by normoxia and hypoxia on cultures of human dermal fibroblasts: How does it affect cell aging? Oxidative Medicine and Cellular Longevity. 2018;**2018**

[107] Sharifi-Rad RYE, Rizk AA, Sadaka C, Zgheib R, Zam W, Zielińska D. Turmeric and its major compound curcumin on health: Bioactive effects and safety profiles for food, pharmaceutical, biotechnological and medicinal applications. Frontiers in Pharmacology. 2020;**11**:01021

[108] Lee W, Loo CY, Bebawy M, Luk F, Mason R, Rohanizadeh R. Curcumin and its derivatives: Their application in neuropharmacology and neuroscience in the 21st century. Current Neuropharmacology. 2013;**11**:338-378. DOI: 10.2174/1570159X11311040002

[109] Priyadarsini KI. The chemistry of curcumin: From extraction to therapeutic agent. Molecules. 2014;**19**(12):20091-20112

[110] Kunnumakkara AB, Hegde M, Parama D, Girisa S, Kumar A,

Daimary UD, et al. Role of turmeric and curcumin in prevention and treatment of chronic diseases: Lessons learned from clinical trials. ACS Pharmacology & Translational Science. 2023;**6**(4):447-518. DOI: 10.1021/Acsptsci.2c00012

[111] Jongrungraungchok S, Madaka F, Wunnakup T, Sudsai T, Pongphaew C, Songsak T, et al. In vitro antioxidant, anti-inflammatory, and anticancer activities of mixture Thai medicinal plants. BMC Complementary Medicine and Therapies. 2023;**23**(1):43

[112] Li P, Pu S, Lin C, He L, Zhao H, Yang C, et al. Curcumin selectively induces colon cancer cell apoptosis and S cell cycle arrest by regulates Rb/E2F/P53 pathway. Journal of Molecular Structure. 2022;**1263**:133180

[113] Lim TG, Lee SY, Huang Z, Lim DY, Chen H, Jung SK, et al. Curcumin suppresses proliferation of colon cancer cells by targeting CDK2. Cancer Prevention Research. 2014;**7**:466-474

[114] Rashad Shimaa E, Abdel-Tawab FM, Fahmy EM, Attalla AG, Ahmed ES, Haggran AA. Determination of genotoxic effects of some food additives on some human cancer cells by flow cytometry analysis. Egyptian Journal of Genetics and Cytology. 2018;**47**:329-343

[115] Ali S, Abdel-Tawab F, Fahmy E, Abodoma A, Rashad S. In vitro assessment of cytotoxic and genotoxic activities of the anticancer drug doxorubicin. Egyptian Journal of Chemistry. 2024;**67**(11):155-167. DOI: 10.21608/ejchem.2023.253832.8963

[116] Rashad SE, Abdel-Tawab FM, Fahmy EM, Attalla AG, Ahmed ES, Haggran AA. Application of the yeast comet assay in testing some food additives for genotoxicity by comet assay in yeast. Egyptian Journal of Chemistry. 2021;**64**(12):7649-7667

[117] Mousa SA, Haggran AA, El-Kawokgy TMA, Abo El-Kheir ZA, Sabry SMH, Rashad SE. Impact assessment of cadmium chloride on human cell lines and yeast knockout strains. Egyptian Pharmaceutical Journal. 2022a;**21**(4)

[118] Mousa SAA, Haggran AEA, El-Kawokgy TM, Abo El-Kheir ZA, Sabry SMH, Rashad SE. Assessment of cytotoxicity and Genotoxicity response of zinc sulphate on eukaryotic cells. Egyptian Journal of Chemistry. 2022b;**65**(11):707-725. DOI: 10.21608/EJCHEM.2022.141668.6209

[119] Rashad SE, Haggran AA, Aboul-Elab EI, Shaalan AH, Abdoon ASS. Cytotoxic and genotoxic effects of 50 nm gold nanorods on mouse splenocytes and human cell lines. Egyptian Journal of Chemistry. 2022;**65**(11):509-514

[120] Bianchi G, Ravera S, Traverso C, Amaro A, Piaggio F, Emionite L, et al. Curcumin induces A fatal energetic impairment in tumor cells in vitro and in vivo by inhibiting ATP-synthase activity. Carcinogenesis. 2018;**39**:1141-1150

[121] Alizadeh M, Kheirouri S. Curcumin reduces malondialdehyde and improves antioxidants in humans with diseased conditions: A comprehensive meta-analysis of randomized controlled trials. Biomedicine. 2019;**9**:4

[122] Chen Y-M, Chiu W-C, Chiu Y-S, Li T, Sung H-C, Hsiao C-Y. Supplementation of nano-bubble curcumin extract improves gut microbiota composition and exercise performance in mice. Food & Function. 2020;**11**(4):3574-3584

[123] Cas DM, Ghidoni R. Dietary curcumin: Correlation between

bioavailability and health potential. Nutrients. 2019;**11**:2147

[124] Kotha RR, Luthria DL. Curcumin: Biological, pharmaceutical, nutraceutical, and analytical aspects. Molecules. 2019;**24**:2930

[125] Nasef NA, Loveday SM, Golding M, Martins RN, Shah TM, Clarke M, et al. Food matrix and co-presence of turmeric compounds influence bioavailability of curcumin in healthy humans. Food & Function. 2019;**10**(8):4584-4592

[126] Hegde M, Girisa S, BharathwajChetty B, Vishwa R, Kunnumakkara AB. Curcumin formulations for better bioavailability: What we learned from clinical trials thus far? ACS Omega. 2023;**8**(12):10713-10746. DOI: 10.1021/acsomega.2c07326

[127] Tang M, Taghibiglou C. The mechanisms of action of curcumin in Alzheimer's disease. Journal of Alzheimer's Disease. 2017;**58**(4):1003-1016. DOI: 10.3233/JAD-170188

[128] She R, Xu P. Mechanism of curcumin in the prevention and treatment of oral submucosal fibrosis and progress in clinical application research. BDJ Open. 2024;**10**:82. DOI: 10.1038/S41405-024-00268-7

[129] Nelson KM, Dahlin JL, Bisson J, et al. The essential medicinal chemistry of curcumin. Journal of Medicinal Chemistry. 2017;**60**(5):1620-1637

[130] Pauli GF, Chen SN, Friesen JB, et al. Analysis and purification of bioactive natural products: The Anapurna study. Journal of Natural Products. 2012;**75**(6):1243-1255

[131] Jennings MR, Parks RJ. Curcumin as an antiviral agent. Viruses. 2020;**12**(11):1242

[132] Nicoliche T, Bartolomeo CS, Lemes RMR, et al. Antiviral, anti-inflammatory and antioxidant effects of curcumin and curcuminoids in SH-SY5Y cells infected by SARS-Cov-2. Scientific Reports. 2024;**14**:10696

[133] Praditya D, Kirchhoff L, Brüning J, Rachmawati H, Steinmann J, Steinmann E. Anti-infective properties of the golden spice curcumin. Frontiers in Microbiology. 2019;**10**:912

[134] Liu S, Liu J, He L, Liu L, Cheng B, Zhou F, et al. A comprehensive review on the benefits and problems of curcumin with respect to human health. Molecules. 2022;**27**(14):4400

Chapter 5

Curcumin in Cancer Therapy: Mechanisms, Delivery Systems, and Clinical Potential

Lubiao Liang and Yajin Zhao

Abstract

Curcumin, a polyphenolic compound derived from the turmeric plant (*Curcuma longa*), has garnered significant attention for its potential anticancer properties due to its ability to modulate multiple molecular targets involved in cancer development and progression. This chapter provides a comprehensive overview of curcumin's mechanisms of action in cancer therapy, focusing on its effects on cell proliferation, apoptosis, metastasis, and inflammation. Curcumin exerts its anticancer effects through various signaling pathways, including the suppression of NF-κB, JAK/STAT3, and PI3K/Akt, and the modulation of cell cycle regulators. Despite its promising anticancer potential, curcumin faces challenges in clinical applications due to its poor bioavailability, low solubility, and rapid metabolism. To overcome these limitations, innovative drug delivery systems, such as nanoparticles, liposomes, and polymer-based formulations, have been developed to enhance curcumin's therapeutic efficacy and stability. These systems improve the solubility, targeted delivery, and controlled release of curcumin, thereby maximizing its anticancer effects while minimizing systemic toxicity. Moreover, preclinical and clinical studies assessing curcumin's clinical potential in combination with other chemotherapeutic agents and its role as an adjuvant in cancer treatment have shown promising results. The chapter concludes by discussing the challenges and future directions of curcumin-based therapies, including the need for further clinical trials to establish optimal dosage, formulation, and therapeutic regimens and the potential for curcumin to be integrated into personalized cancer treatments.

Keywords: curcumin, cancer therapy, mechanisms of action, drug delivery systems, clinical translation

1. Introduction

Curcumin, a bioactive polyphenol derived from *Curcuma longa* L. rhizomes, has gained significant attention for its potent anticancer properties. Extensive research has demonstrated its ability to modulate multiple oncogenic pathways, including inhibition of tumor cell proliferation [1], induction of apoptosis [2], suppression of inflammation [3, 4], and prevention of metastasis [5, 6]. These multifaceted mechanisms make curcumin a promising candidate for cancer prevention and therapy. Preclinical studies have shown its efficacy against various malignancies, including breast [7, 8], lung [9], colorectal [10], pancreatic [11–14], prostate [15, 16], ovarian [17, 18], hepatocellular [19, 20], head and neck cancers [21, 22], leukemia [23], and myeloma [24].

Despite its therapeutic potential, the clinical translation of curcumin remains challenging due to its poor aqueous solubility [25–27], rapid metabolism [28, 29], low bioavailability [30], and limited tissue penetration [31, 32]. These pharmacokinetic limitations significantly hinder its efficacy in cancer treatment. To address these challenges, advanced curcumin delivery systems (CDSs) have been developed, including nanoparticles [31], co-amorphous formulations [30], cyclodextrin encapsulation [33], solid dispersions, and nanosuspensions [34], which aim to enhance curcumin's solubility, stability, and targeted delivery.

This chapter provides a comprehensive review of curcumin's role in cancer therapy, focusing on its molecular mechanisms, innovative drug delivery strategies, and clinical potential. By exploring recent advancements in CDSs, we highlight how these formulations can overcome existing barriers, optimize curcumin's therapeutic efficacy, and pave the way for its integration into modern oncological treatments.

2. Mechanisms of action in cancer therapy

2.1 Effects on cell cycle and cell proliferation

Curcumin exerts its anticancer effects through multiple mechanisms that target various stages of cancer progression, including tumor proliferation, cell cycle regulation, angiogenesis, and metastasis [35–38]. One of the key ways curcumin inhibits cancer development is by disrupting tumor cell proliferation and inducing cell cycle arrest. Curcumin has been shown to influence the expression of cyclins, cyclin-dependent kinases (CDKs), and cell cycle regulators, leading to the inhibition of G1/S phase transition [39]. Furthermore, curcumin inhibits the proliferation of lung cancer and cervical cancer cells by downregulating cyclin D1 and upregulating cyclin B1 in the TGF-β pathway, further downregulating Ki67 and inhibiting proliferating cell nuclear antigen overexpression and resulting in cell cycle arrest [40–44]. By halting the progression of the cell cycle, curcumin effectively prevents the uncontrolled cell division characteristic of tumors.

2.2 Induction of apoptosis

In addition to its effects on the cell cycle, curcumin modulates several critical signaling pathways that play a central role in tumorigenesis [45]. One of the most significant pathways is NF-κB (nuclear factor kappa-light-chain-enhancer of activated B cells), which regulates inflammation, cell survival, and immune responses [46]. Curcumin inhibits NF-κB activation, thereby reducing the expression of pro-inflammatory cytokines and inhibiting tumor growth and survival [37, 47–49]. B-cell lymphoma protein 2 (Bcl-2), an antiapoptotic protein inhibiting pro-apoptotic factors like Bax, caspase 8, and caspase 3/7 or 9, is impacted by curcumin. It is found that curcumin can downregulate Bcl-2 and upregulate Bax, promoting the activation of caspases and poly-ADP ribose polymerase (PARP), ultimately facilitating caspase-dependent cell death, including osteosarcoma [42], breast cancer [33], and HeLa cancer cells [50]. Additionally, curcumin suppresses cell proliferation and triggers apoptosis in vemurafenib-resistant melanoma cells by downregulating the EGFR signaling pathway [51, 52], highlighting its potential to overcome drug resistance.

2.3 Effects on cell invasion and metastasis

Curcumin can inhibit multifaceted inhibitory effects on cancer invasion and metastasis by modulating key signaling pathways. Specifically, they suppress the TGF-β/Smad3 signaling pathway, leading to the downregulating NF-κB signaling pathway, impacting inflammatory and immune responses. NF-κB, in turn, regulates pivotal genes such as B lymphoma Mo-MLV insertion region 1 (BMI1), phosphatase and tensin homolog deleted on chromosome ten (PTEN), and components involved in epithelial-mesenchymal transition (EMT), influencing tumor genesis and progression [39, 41, 43, 47]. By inhibiting the Wnt/β-catenin pathway, curcumin reduces cancer stem cell characteristics and decreases tumor growth and metastasis [49, 53]. Similarly, curcumin interferes with the JAK/STAT3 signaling pathway, which is often constitutively activated in various cancers and contributes to tumorigenesis, immune evasion, and resistance to therapy [54]. By suppressing JAK/STAT3 signaling, curcumin promotes apoptosis and inhibits cancer cell proliferation [55, 56].

Moreover, curcumin exerts antiangiogenic effects by inhibiting the formation of new blood vessels that supply nutrients to tumors, a critical process in cancer progression. It also suppresses the invasion and metastasis of cancer cells by downregulating the expression of various matrix metalloproteinases (MMPs), including MMP-2 [57], MMP-9 [58, 59], and MMP-10 [60], which has been observed in different cancer types, such as tongue carcinoma, lung cancer, oral squamous cell carcinoma, and hepatocellular carcinoma. And curcumin affects several signaling pathways that regulate MMP expression and cancer cell invasion. It inhibits pathways such as Rac1/PAK1 [61], ERK/NF-κB [62], and PKCα [63], which are involved in the regulation of MMPs and other proteins that facilitate cancer cell migration and invasion. By modulating these signaling pathways, curcumin effectively impedes multiple aspects of cancer biology, making it a powerful agent in cancer therapy.

2.4 Enhancement of chemotherapy and radiotherapy

Curcumin has been shown to increase the effectiveness of chemotherapy and radiotherapy by sensitizing tumor cells, thereby improving patient survival times and reducing tumor growth and metastasis [48, 64–66]. When used in combination with chemotherapeutic drugs like doxorubicin, paclitaxel, and cisplatin, curcumin enhances their anticancer efficacy by modulating various molecular pathways and reducing drug resistance [67–69].

Moreover, curcumin's anti-inflammatory and antioxidant properties help alleviate chemotherapy- and radiotherapy-induced side effects, including dermatitis, mucositis, and other inflammatory reactions. Its anti-inflammatory activity is primarily mediated through the inhibition of NF-κB signaling, leading to a reduction in pro-inflammatory cytokine production and oxidative stress [65, 70, 71].

3. Advances in curcumin delivery system

One of the major challenges in the clinical use of curcumin for cancer therapy is its poor bioavailability due to its low solubility, rapid metabolism, and systemic elimination. To overcome these limitations, significant progress has been made in the development of innovative curcumin delivery systems (CDSs) designed to improve curcumin's therapeutic efficacy [72]. These systems utilize various carrier technologies, such as nanoparticles, micelles, and hydrogels, to enhance curcumin's solubility, stability, and targeted delivery to cancer cells.

Nanoparticles are a prominent method for curcumin delivery, offering improved bioavailability and targeted delivery. Magnetic alginate/chitosan nanoparticles have been shown to enhance the uptake efficiency and cytotoxicity of curcumin in breast cancer cells, with a three- to sixfold increase in uptake compared to free curcumin [73]. Similarly, hyaluronic acid-modified mesoporous silica nanoparticles have demonstrated increased anticancer efficacy by targeting CD-44 receptors in cancer cells [74]. Metal-polyphenol networks also provide a stable and efficient delivery system, enhancing curcumin's anticancer activity [75]. These nanoparticles can be engineered to target specific tumor cells, thereby enhancing curcumin's local concentration at the site of action while minimizing systemic toxicity. Hydrogels, which are three-dimensional networks of hydrophilic polymers, also offer a promising approach for sustained and localized curcumin delivery. Hydrogels have demonstrated high encapsulation efficiencies for curcumin, with some formulations achieving nearly 100% encapsulation [76, 77].

Folate-modified curcumin-loaded micelles have been developed to improve solubility and anticancer activity. These micelles show enhanced cytotoxicity and cellular uptake in cancer cells, with a threefold increase in half-life compared to solubilized curcumin [78]. Other innovative systems include dextran-based nanosized carriers for liver cancer targeting, which offer controlled and targeted delivery with high toxicity toward hepatic cells [79]. Microbubble-mediated delivery systems, when combined with ultrasound, significantly enhance curcumin uptake and reduce cell viability in cervical cancer cells [80].

The use of these CDSs offers several benefits, including enhanced bioavailability, improved stability, and the ability to achieve targeted delivery, which collectively increase curcumin's therapeutic efficacy. These systems also enable the reduction of side effects associated with curcumin's systemic administration, making it a more viable option for cancer therapy.

Emerging technologies are further enhancing the potential of CDSs for curcumin delivery. For instance, carbon dots derived from fruit peels have been used to enhance curcumin's antimicrobial and antioxidant activities, offering a novel approach to improve its bioavailability [81]. Additionally, block copolymers and polycyclodextrins have been used to significantly increase curcumin's solubility and provide controlled release, enhancing its therapeutic potential [82].

Overall, these advances in curcumin delivery systems represent a significant step forward in making curcumin a more effective and clinically applicable agent in cancer therapy.

4. Preclinical and clinical applications of curcumin

4.1 Key preclinical studies demonstrating anticancer effects

Curcumin, a natural compound derived from the turmeric plant, has been extensively studied in preclinical models for its potential anticancer effects. Key studies have demonstrated that curcumin can inhibit cancer cell proliferation, induce apoptosis (programmed cell death) [33, 42, 50], and suppress metastasis [39, 41, 43, 47, 49, 53]. Through its multifaceted mechanisms, curcumin interacts with various signaling pathways involved in cancer development, such as the NF-κB [3], TGF-β [6, 40], and Wnt/β-catenin pathways [37, 47–49]. These pathways regulate critical processes like inflammation, cell growth, and metastasis. Studies also indicate that curcumin can modulate the expression of key regulatory molecules, including microRNAs and long non-coding RNAs, which are involved in tumorigenesis [35, 45]. Additionally, curcumin has shown promise in reversing multidrug resistance in cancer cells by down-regulating P-glycoprotein (P-gp), a key player in chemotherapy resistance, thereby improving the efficacy of chemotherapy drugs [83, 84]. Furthermore, curcumin's potential to influence the tumor microenvironment by reducing inflammation and immune suppression has been observed. By modulating immune responses, curcumin enhances the effectiveness of immune-based cancer therapies, making it a valuable adjunct to cancer treatment [85, 86].

4.2 Clinical trials evaluating safety, tolerability, and efficacy

Clinical trials evaluating curcumin's role in cancer therapy have underscored its potential as a safe and effective agent. Several studies have investigated curcumin delivery systems (CDSs) designed to enhance curcumin's bioavailability and therapeutic effects. These systems aim to improve curcumin's pharmacokinetics, protect it from degradation, and increase its cellular uptake, addressing the challenge of curcumin's poor bioavailability in its natural form.

A search of the World Health Organization International Clinical Trials Registry Platform (ICTRP) identified a total of 75 clinical trials investigating curcumin in cancer therapy, with six specifically focusing on curcumin drug delivery systems (CDSs) [72]. These trials have primarily targeted breast, colon, prostate, and advanced/metastatic cancers, highlighting the growing interest in curcumin's potential in cancer treatment. For instance, a Phase 1 dose-escalation study evaluated curcumin liposomes in cancer patients, demonstrating the safety and tolerability of curcumin at doses ranging from 100 to 300 mg/m^2 with no dose-limiting toxicity observed [87]. Promising reductions in tumor markers were noted in patients with prostate [15], colon [88], and metastatic cancers [87]. A Randomized Double-Blind Placebo-Controlled Phase IIB Trial of curcumin in oral leukoplakia found that curcumin (3.6 g/day for 6 months) is a well-tolerated and demonstrated significant and durable clinical response for oral leukoplakia, with no safety concerns [89]. Oral curcumin, 6.0 g daily during radiotherapy, reduced the severity of radiation dermatitis in breast cancer patients [7]. Curcumin can decrease aberrant crypt foci number in colorectal cancer patients, potentially mediated by curcumin conjugates delivered systemically [88]. Oral curcumin is well-tolerated and shows biological activity in some advanced pancreatic cancer patients despite limited absorption [14]. These findings suggest that curcumin, when properly formulated, is well-tolerated and offers therapeutic benefits in reducing tumor burden.

4.3 Potential as an adjuvant in chemotherapy and radiotherapy

Curcumin has shown considerable promise as an adjuvant in combination with chemotherapy and radiotherapy [48, 64–66]. In preclinical studies, curcumin enhances the sensitivity of cancer cells to chemotherapy drugs by downregulating key resistance mechanisms, such as P-gp expression, ATP activity, and cancer stem cell populations, thereby reversing multidrug resistance and increasing the efficacy of chemotherapeutic agents [83, 84, 90, 91]. This synergistic effect makes curcumin an attractive candidate for use alongside conventional chemotherapy, as it may increase the effectiveness of treatment while reducing the likelihood of resistance.

Additionally, curcumin's anti-inflammatory and antioxidant properties can improve the therapeutic outcomes of radiotherapy. By modulating the tumor microenvironment, curcumin reduces oxidative stress and inflammation, which are often exacerbated by radiation therapy [65]. This may mitigate the side effects of radiotherapy, enhance tumor response, and improve overall patient outcomes [70].

Overall, curcumin's potential as an adjunct to chemotherapy and radiotherapy offers a promising strategy to improve cancer treatment outcomes, reduce side effects, and overcome resistance to standard therapies.

5. Challenges in clinical translation

5.1 Issues with bioavailability, dosing regimens, and variability in results

One of the major challenges in the clinical translation of curcumin is its low bioavailability [92, 93]. Curcumin exhibits poor water solubility, rapid metabolism, and limited systemic absorption, which significantly reduces its therapeutic potential when administered orally in its natural form. As a result, achieving effective therapeutic concentrations of curcumin in the body is difficult, and the results of clinical studies are often inconsistent.

Dosing regimens also pose a challenge [94, 95]. The optimal dose of curcumin for cancer therapy is still under investigation, and variability in dosing protocols across studies has led to inconsistent outcomes. Different formulations, delivery methods, and dosing schedules complicate the interpretation of results, making it difficult to determine the most effective approach for clinical use.

Moreover, the variability in results across clinical trials is another significant issue. Despite promising preclinical data, many clinical trials have reported limited efficacy or inconclusive results. This could be attributed to factors such as variations in patient populations, tumor types, and treatment regimens, as well as the inherent complexities of curcumin's pharmacokinetics.

6. Future directions in curcumin-based cancer therapies

6.1 Role of gut microbiota in curcumin metabolism and efficacy

Emerging research suggests that the gut microbiota plays a crucial role in the metabolism and efficacy of curcumin [96–98]. The gut microbiome influences the bioavailability of curcumin through enzymatic modification, which can either enhance or reduce its therapeutic potential [99]. Certain gut bacteria are capable of metabolizing curcumin into bioactive metabolites, which may have different pharmacological activities compared to the parent compound.

Understanding the interaction between curcumin and the gut microbiota could lead to personalized approaches in curcumin-based therapies, optimizing its therapeutic efficacy. Manipulating the gut microbiome through prebiotics, probiotics, or dietary modifications might enhance curcumin's absorption and increase its anticancer properties. This could also help overcome some of the challenges related to curcumin's poor bioavailability and variability in clinical outcomes.

Future studies should focus on identifying specific microbiota species that facilitate curcumin metabolism and understanding how they influence curcumin's anticancer effects. This knowledge could lead to the development of microbiome-targeted strategies to improve the effectiveness of curcumin in cancer treatment.

6.2 Exploration of curcumin's role in immunomodulation and drug resistance reversal

Curcumin's potential as an immunomodulator in cancer therapy is an exciting avenue for future research [36]. Curcumin has been shown to influence immune cell activity, including promoting the activation of T cells, natural killer (NK) cells, and macrophages, while inhibiting the function of immunosuppressive cells such as regulatory T cells (Tregs) [5]. This ability to modulate the immune system could enhance the effectiveness of immunotherapies, making curcumin a valuable adjunct in cancer treatment.

Additionally, curcumin's role in reversing drug resistance is an important area of investigation [100]. Drug resistance remains a major challenge in cancer therapy, particularly in relation to chemotherapeutic agents. Curcumin has demonstrated the ability to modulate key signaling pathways involved in drug resistance, including those related to the P-gp pump and the EMT. By restoring sensitivity to chemotherapy drugs and overcoming resistance mechanisms, curcumin could improve the success of conventional therapies and reduce the need for high-dose treatments.

Further research is required to elucidate the precise molecular mechanisms by which curcumin modulates immune responses and reverses drug resistance. This could lead to the development of curcumin-based combination therapies that enhance the effectiveness of both immune-based and conventional cancer treatments.

7. Conclusion

Curcumin, a natural polyphenolic compound derived from the turmeric plant, has demonstrated significant potential as a transformative agent in cancer therapy. Its multifaceted biological activities, including anti-inflammatory, antioxidant, anticancer, and immunomodulatory effects, make it a promising candidate for the development of novel cancer treatments. Curcumin's ability to modulate critical cellular signaling pathways involved in cancer cell proliferation, invasion, metastasis, and resistance to therapy, positions it as an adjunct or even a complementary treatment in combination with traditional cancer therapies.

Moreover, curcumin's versatile delivery systems, such as curcumin drug delivery systems (CDSs), have addressed key challenges related to its poor bioavailability, enhancing its therapeutic potential in clinical settings. Preclinical and early-stage clinical studies have shown promising results, suggesting that curcumin can reduce tumor growth and metastasis and improve the efficacy of chemotherapy and radiotherapy while minimizing associated side effects.

However, despite these encouraging findings, several challenges remain in translating curcumin's therapeutic potential into routine clinical practice. Issues such as its bioavailability, optimal dosing regimens, and variability in treatment responses need to be addressed. Further research is crucial to refine curcumin formulations, explore its synergistic combinations with other therapies, and develop more effective delivery methods.

The role of curcumin in overcoming cancer-related challenges, such as drug resistance and immune suppression, as well as its applications in innovative therapies like photothermal and imaging-guided treatments, highlights its transformative potential. However, to fully realize its clinical promise, there is an urgent need for extensive clinical trials that evaluate its safety, efficacy, and long-term effects in diverse patient populations.

In conclusion, while curcumin has emerged as a powerful therapeutic agent with substantial promise, its full integration into cancer treatment regimens will require continued research, optimization of its delivery, and rigorous clinical validation. With further advancements, curcumin could become a cornerstone of cancer therapy, providing patients with more effective and less toxic treatment options.

Acknowledgements

This work was supported by the National Natural Science Foundation of China (No. 32060220) and the Natural Science and Technology Foundation of Guizhou (No. QKH [2020]1Y094). The authors acknowledge the use of ChatGPT 4o Mini for language polishing of the manuscript.

Conflict of interest

The authors declare no conflict of interest.

Author details

Lubiao Liang[1,2] and Yajin Zhao[1,2]*

1 Department of Oral Pathology, School/Hospital of Stomatology, Zunyi Medical University, Zunyi, Guizhou, China

2 Department of Thoracis Surgery, Affiliated Hospital of Zunyi Medical University, Zunyi, Guizhou, China

*Address all correspondence to: zhaoyajinyy@163.com

References

[1] Kunnumakkara AB, Anand P, Aggarwal BB. Curcumin inhibits proliferation, invasion, angiogenesis and metastasis of different cancers through interaction with multiple cell signaling proteins. Cancer Letters. 2008;**269**(2):199-225

[2] Moustapha A et al. Curcumin induces crosstalk between autophagy and apoptosis mediated by calcium release from the endoplasmic reticulum, lysosomal destabilization and mitochondrial events. Cell Death Discovery. 2015;**1**:15017

[3] Cho J-W, Lee K-S, Kim C-W. Curcumin attenuates the expression of IL-1beta, IL-6, and TNF-alpha as well as cyclin E in TNF-alpha-treated HaCaT cells; NF-kappaB and MAPKs as potential upstream targets. International Journal of Molecular Medicine. 2007;**19**(3):469-474

[4] Panahi Y et al. Adjuvant therapy with bioavailability-boosted curcuminoids suppresses systemic inflammation and improves quality of life in patients with solid tumors: A randomized double-blind placebo-controlled trial. Phytotherapy Research. 2014;**28**(10):1461-1467

[5] James MI et al. Curcumin inhibits cancer stem cell phenotypes in ex vivo models of colorectal liver metastases, and is clinically safe and tolerable in combination with FOLFOX chemotherapy. Cancer Letters. 2015;**364**(2):135-141

[6] Kunihiro AG et al. Curcumin, but not curcumin-glucuronide, inhibits Smad signaling in TGFbeta-dependent bone metastatic breast cancer cells and is enriched in bone compared to other tissues. The Journal of Nutritional Biochemistry. 2019;**63**:150-156

[7] Ryan JL et al. Curcumin for radiation dermatitis: A randomized, double-blind, placebo-controlled clinical trial of thirty breast cancer patients. Radiation Research. 2013;**180**(1):34-43

[8] Bayet-Robert M et al. Phase I dose escalation trial of docetaxel plus curcumin in patients with advanced and metastatic breast cancer. Cancer Biology & Therapy. 2010;**9**(1):8-14

[9] Alexandrow MG et al. Curcumin: A novel Stat3 pathway inhibitor for chemoprevention of lung cancer. European Journal of Cancer Prevention. 2012;**21**(5):407-412

[10] Howells LM et al. Curcumin combined with FOLFOX chemotherapy is safe and tolerable in patients with metastatic colorectal cancer in a randomized phase IIa trial. The Journal of Nutrition. 2019;**149**(7):1133-1139

[11] Masashi Kanai KY, Asada M, Imaizumi A, Suzuki C, Matsumoto S, Nishimura T, et al. A phase I: II study of gemcitabine-based chemotherapy plus curcumin for patients with gemcitabine-resistant pancreatic cancer. Cancer Chemotherapy and Pharmacology. 2011;**68**(1):157-164

[12] Pastorelli D, Giovanis P, et al. Phytosome complex of curcumin as complementary therapy of advanced pancreatic cancer improves safety and efficacy of gemcitabine: Results of a prospective phase II trial. Pharmacological Research. 2018;**132**:72-79

[13] Epelbaum R et al. Curcumin and gemcitabine in patients with advanced pancreatic cancer. Nutrition and Cancer. 2010;**62**(8):1137-1141

[14] Dhillon N et al. Phase II trial of curcumin in patients with advanced pancreatic cancer. Clinical Cancer Research. 2008;**14**(14):4491-4499

[15] Passildas-Jahanmohan J et al. Multicenter randomized phase II study comparing docetaxel plus curcumin versus docetaxel plus placebo in first-line treatment of metastatic castration-resistant prostate cancer. Cancer Medicine. 2021;**10**(7):2332-2340

[16] Jalal Hejazi RR, Taleban F-A, Molana S-H, Hejazi E, Ehtejab G, Hara N. Effect of curcumin supplementation during radiotherapy on oxidative status of patients with prostate cancer: A double blinded, randomized, placebo-controlled study. Nutrition and Cancer. 2016;**68**(1):77-85

[17] Lin YG et al. Curcumin inhibits tumor growth and angiogenesis in ovarian carcinoma by targeting the nuclear factor-kappaB pathway. Clinical Cancer Research. 2007;**13**(11):3423-3430

[18] Barinda AJ et al. Curcumin prevents epithelial-to mesenchymal transition-mediated ovarian cancer progression through NRF2/ETBR/ET-1 Axis and preserves mitochondria biogenesis in kidney after cisplatin administration. Advanced Pharmaceutical Bulletin. 2022;**12**(1):128-141

[19] Moordiani M et al. Curcumin analogs PGV-1 and CCA-1.1 induce cell cycle arrest in human hepatocellular carcinoma cells with overexpressed MYCN. The Indonesian Biomedical Journal. 2023;**15**(2):141-149

[20] Li Y et al. Protective role of curcumin in disease progression from non-alcoholic fatty liver disease to hepatocellular carcinoma: A meta-analysis. Frontiers in Pharmacology. 2024;**15**:1343193

[21] Delavarian Z et al. Oral administration of nanomicelle curcumin in the prevention of radiotherapy-induced mucositis in head and neck cancers. Special Care in Dentistry. 2019;**39**(2):166-172

[22] Arun P, Sagayaraj A, Azeem Mohiyuddin SM, Santosh D. Role of turmeric extract in minimising mucositis in patients receiving radiotherapy for head and neck squamous cell cancer: A randomised, placebo-controlled trial. The Journal of Laryngology and Otology. 7 Feb 2020:1-6. DOI: 10.1017/S0022215120000316

[23] Ghalaut VS et al. Effect of imatinib therapy with and without turmeric powder on nitric oxide levels in chronic myeloid leukemia. Journal of Oncology Pharmacy Practice. 2012;**18**(2):186-190

[24] Zaidi A, Lai M, Cavenagh J. Long-term stabilisation of myeloma with curcumin. BMJ Case Reports. 2017;**2017**:bcr2016218148

[25] Stanić Z. Curcumin, a compound from natural sources, a true scientific challenge—A review. Plant Foods for Human Nutrition. 2017;**72**:1-12

[26] Mohanty C, Das M, Sahoo S. Emerging role of nanocarriers to increase the solubility and bioavailability of curcumin. Expert Opinion on Drug Delivery. 2012;**9**:1347-1364

[27] Ziwei Ma NW, He H, Tang X. Pharmaceutical strategies of improving oral systemic bioavailability of curcumin for clinical application. Journal of Controlled Release: Official Journal of the Controlled Release Society. 2019;**28**(316):359-380

[28] Wahlang B, Bansal A. Identification of permeability-related hurdles in oral delivery of curcumin using the

Caco-2 cell model. European Journal of Pharmaceutics and Biopharmaceutics. 2011;**77**(2):275-282

[29] Dei Cas M, Ghidoni R. Dietary curcumin: Correlation between bioavailability and health potential. Nutrients. 2019;**11**(9):2147

[30] Ruoning Wang JH, Jiang A, Huang R, Fu T, Wang L, Zheng Q, et al. Involvement of metabolism-permeability in enhancing the oral bioavailability of curcumin in excipient-free solid dispersions co-formed with piperine. International Journal of Pharmaceutics. 2019;**561**:9-18

[31] Kanwal Q et al. Curcumin nanoparticles: Physicochemical fabrication, characterization, antioxidant, enzyme inhibition, molecular docking and simulation studies. RSC Advances. 2023;**13**(32):22268-22280

[32] Stohs SJ et al. Highly bioavailable forms of curcumin and promising avenues for curcumin-based research and application: A review. Molecules. 2020;**25**(6):1397

[33] Low ZX et al. Biophysical evaluation of water-soluble curcumin encapsulated in beta-Cyclodextrins on colorectal cancer cells. International Journal of Molecular Sciences. 2022;**23**(21):12866

[34] Aditya N, Kim S, Ko S. Fabrication of amorphous curcumin nanosuspensions using β-lactoglobulin to enhance solubility, stability, and bioavailability. Colloids and Surfaces B: Biointerfaces. 2015;**127**:114-121

[35] Abd Wahab NA et al. Mechanism of anti-cancer activity of curcumin on androgen-dependent and androgen-independent prostate cancer. Nutrients. 2020;**12**(3):679

[36] Giordano A, Tommonaro G. Curcumin and cancer. Nutrients. 2019;**11**(10):2376

[37] Ashrafizadeh M, Makvandi P, Zarrabi A, Farkhondeh T, Samarghandian S. Versatile role of curcumin and its derivatives in lung cancer therapy. Journal of Cellular Physiology. 2020;**235**:9241-9268

[38] Zoi V et al. The role of curcumin in cancer treatment. Biomedicine. 2021;**9**(9):1086

[39] Liu J et al. LncRNA NR2F2-AS1 silencing induces cell cycle arrest in G0/G1 phase via downregulating cyclin D1 in colorectal cancer. Cancer Management and Research. 2020;**12**:1835-1843

[40] Shariati M et al. Nanocurcumin-mediated down-regulation of telomerase via stimulating TGFbeta1 signaling pathway in hepatocellular carcinoma cells. Iranian Biomedical Journal. 2018;**22**(3):171-179

[41] Zaman MS et al. Curcumin nanoformulation for cervical cancer treatment. Scientific Reports. 2016;**6**:20051

[42] Dhule SS et al. The combined effect of encapsulating curcumin and C6 ceramide in liposomal nanoparticles against osteosarcoma. Molecular Pharmaceutics. 2014;**11**(2):417-427

[43] Vijayakurup V et al. Chitosan encapsulation enhances the bioavailability and tissue retention of curcumin and improves its efficacy in preventing B[a]P-induced lung carcinogenesis. Cancer Prevention Research (Philadelphia, Pa.). 2019;**12**(4):225-236

[44] Mortezaee K, Mirtavoos-Mahyari H, Motevaseli E, Najafi M, Farhood B, Rosengren R, et al. Mechanisms of apoptosis modulation by curcumin:

Implications for cancer therapy. Journal of Cellular Physiology. 2019;**234**(8):12537-12550

[45] Wang M et al. Potential mechanisms of action of curcumin for cancer prevention: Focus on cellular signaling pathways and miRNAs. International Journal of Biological Sciences. 2019;**15**(6):1200-1214

[46] Pavitra E et al. The role of NF-kappaB in breast cancer initiation, growth, metastasis, and resistance to chemotherapy. Biomedicine & Pharmacotherapy. 2023;**163**:114822

[47] Mahjoub MA, Babak B, Sadeghizadeh M, Babashah S. Combination treatment with dendrosomal nanocurcumin and doxorubicin improves anticancer effects on breast cancer cells through modulating CXCR4/NF-kappaB/Smo regulatory network. Molecular Biology Reports. 2017;**44**(4):341-351

[48] Tan BL, Norhaizan ME. Curcumin combination chemotherapy: The implication and efficacy in cancer. Molecules. 2019;**24**(14):2527

[49] Ghasemi F et al. Curcumin inhibits NF-kB and Wnt/beta-catenin pathways in cervical cancer cells. Pathology, Research and Practice. 2019;**215**(10):152556

[50] Ahmadi F et al. Induction of apoptosis in HeLa cancer cells by an ultrasonic-mediated synthesis of curcumin-loaded chitosan-alginate-STPP nanoparticles. International Journal of Nanomedicine. 2017;**12**:8545-8556

[51] Saeideh Jafarinejad-Farsangi MSH, Rouholamini SEY, Gharbi S, Ansari-Asl Z, Jafari E, Dezfuli AS, et al. Curcumin loaded on graphene nanosheets induced cell death in mammospheres from MCF-7 and primary breast tumor cells. Biomedical Materials. 2021;**16**:045040

[52] Yu-Jen Chiu J-SY, Tsai F-J, Chiu H-Y, Juan Y-N, Lo Y-H, Chiang J-H. Curcumin suppresses cell proliferation and triggers apoptosis in vemurafenib-resistant melanoma cells by downregulating the EGFR signaling pathway. Environmental Toxicology. 2022;**37**(4):868-879

[53] Liu J et al. Wnt/beta-catenin signalling: Function, biological mechanisms, and therapeutic opportunities. Signal Transduction and Targeted Therapy. 2022;**7**(1):3

[54] Chen S et al. Tumor-associated macrophages promote migration and invasion via modulating IL-6/STAT3 signaling in renal cell carcinoma. International Immunopharmacology. 2022;**111**:109139

[55] Khan AQ et al. Curcumin-mediated apoptotic cell death in papillary thyroid cancer and cancer stem-like cells through targeting of the JAK/STAT3 signaling pathway. International Journal of Molecular Sciences. 2020;**21**(2):438

[56] Sandhiutami NMD et al. Curcumin nanoparticle enhances the anticancer effect of cisplatin by inhibiting PI3K/AKT and JAK/STAT3 pathway in rat ovarian carcinoma induced by DMBA. Frontiers in Pharmacology. 2020;**11**:603235

[57] Lee AY et al. Curcumin inhibits invasiveness and epithelial-mesenchymal transition in oral squamous cell carcinoma through reducing matrix metalloproteinase 2, 9 and modulating p53-E-cadherin pathway. Integrative Cancer Therapies. 2015;**14**(5):484-490

[58] Yodkeeree S et al. Curcumin, demethoxycurcumin and bisdemethoxycurcumin differentially

inhibit cancer cell invasion through the down-regulation of MMPs and uPA. The Journal of Nutritional Biochemistry. 2009;**20**(2):87-95

[59] Lin SS et al. Curcumin inhibits the migration and invasion of human A549 lung cancer cells through the inhibition of matrix metalloproteinase-2 and -9 and vascular endothelial growth factor (VEGF). Cancer Letters. 2009;**285**(2):127-133

[60] Tsang RK-Y, Whitney Wing-Yan T, Gao W, Ho W-K, Chan JY-W, Wei WI, et al. Curcumin inhibits tongue carcinoma cells migration and invasion through downregulation of matrix metallopeptidase 10. Cancer Investigation. 2012;**30**(7):503-512

[61] Chen QY et al. Curcumin inhibits lung cancer cell migration and invasion through Rac1-dependent signaling pathway. The Journal of Nutritional Biochemistry. 2014;**25**(2):177-185

[62] Cao L et al. Curcumin inhibits H_2O_2-induced invasion and migration of human pancreatic cancer via suppression of the ERK/NF-kappaB pathway. Oncology Reports. 2016;**36**(4):2245-2251

[63] Kim JM et al. Curcumin suppresses the TPA-induced invasion through inhibition of PKCalpha-dependent MMP-expression in MCF-7 human breast cancer cells. Phytomedicine. 2012;**19**(12):1085-1092

[64] Mansouri K et al. Clinical effects of curcumin in enhancing cancer therapy: A systematic review. BMC Cancer. 2020;**20**(1):791

[65] Bagher Farhood KM, Goradel NH, Khanlarkhani N, Salehi E, Nashtaei MS, Najafi M, et al. Curcumin as an anti-inflammatory agent: Implications to radiotherapy and chemotherapy. Journal of Cellular Physiology. 2020;**234**(5):5728-5740

[66] Farghadani R, Naidu R. Curcumin as an enhancer of therapeutic efficiency of chemotherapy drugs in breast cancer. International Journal of Molecular Sciences. 2022;**23**(4):2144

[67] Ashrafizadeh M et al. Curcumin in cancer therapy: A novel adjunct for combination chemotherapy with paclitaxel and alleviation of its adverse effects. Life Sciences. 2020;**256**:117984

[68] Younes M et al. The synergistic effects of curcumin and chemotherapeutic drugs in inhibiting metastatic, invasive and proliferative pathways. Plants (Basel). 2022;**11**(16):2137

[69] Najafi M et al. The role of curcumin/curcuminoids during gastric cancer chemotherapy: A systematic review of non-clinical study. Life Sciences. 2020;**257**:118051

[70] Akbari S, Elnaz K, Jannati M, Elyasi S, Tayarani-Najaran Z. Curcumin as a preventive or therapeutic measure for chemotherapy and radiotherapy induced adverse reaction: A comprehensive review. Food and Chemical Toxicology. 2020;**145**:111699

[71] Yang Q et al. Effect of curcumin extract against oxidative stress on both structure and deformation capability of red blood cell. Journal of Biomechanics. 2019;**95**:109301

[72] Wang Y, Liang L, Zhao Y. Curcumin delivery systems: How far from clinical application in tumor therapy? Natural Product Communications. 2024;**19**(2):1-13

[73] Song W et al. Magnetic alginate/chitosan nanoparticles for targeted delivery of curcumin into human breast

cancer cells. Nanomaterials (Basel). 2018;**8**(11):907

[74] Shatadal Ghosh SD, Sarkar A, Mousumi K, Sil P. Targeted delivery of curcumin in breast cancer cells via hyaluronic acid modified mesoporous silica nanoparticle to enhance anticancer efficiency. Colloids and Surfaces B: Biointerfaces. 2021;**197**:111404

[75] Yuanyuan Chen DJ, Wang Q, Yueru Sun Z, Rao XL, Ji-chun Zhao K, Zeng ZX, et al. Promotion of the anticancer activity of curcumin based on a metal-polyphenol networks delivery system. International Journal of Pharmaceutics. 2021;**602**(1):120650

[76] Ning P et al. High encapsulation and localized delivery of curcumin from an injectable hydrogel. Materials Science & Engineering. C, Materials for Biological Applications. 2018;**83**:121-129

[77] Dhanya George PUM, Begum KMMS. Chitosan-cellulose hydrogel conjugated with L-histidine and zinc oxide nanoparticles for sustained drug delivery: Kinetics and *in-vitro* biological studies. Carbohydrate Polymers. 2020;**236**(15):116101

[78] Yang C, Hao C, Zhao J, Pang X, Xi Y, Zhai G. Development of a folate-modified curcumin loaded micelle delivery system for cancer targeting. Colloids and Surfaces B: Biointerfaces. 2014;**121**(1):106-113

[79] Anirudhan B. TS. Dextran based nanosized carrier for the controlled and targeted delivery of curcumin to liver cancer cells. International Journal of Biological Macromolecules. 2016;**88**:222-235

[80] Upadhyay A et al. Microbubble-mediated enhanced delivery of curcumin to cervical cancer cells. ACS Omega. 2018;**3**(10):12824-12831

[81] Patel PJ, Shilpa G, Naik R, Kailasa SK, Jha S, Patel SB, et al. Fruit Peel derived carbon dots for improved curcumin delivery: A promising strategy for enhanced antimicrobial and antioxidant activity. ChemistrySelect. 2024;**9**(32):e202400762

[82] Nagy NZ et al. Highly enhanced curcumin delivery applying association type nanostructures of block copolymers, cyclodextrins and polycyclodextrins. Polymers (Basel). 2020;**12**(9):2167

[83] Lopes-Rodrigues V et al. A novel curcumin derivative which inhibits P-glycoprotein, arrests cell cycle and induces apoptosis in multidrug resistance cells. Bioorganic & Medicinal Chemistry. 2017;**25**(2):581-596

[84] Attia YM, Dina ME-K, Ammar RA, Adel A, Khalil A, Walid H, et al. Inhibition of aldehyde dehydrogenase-1 and p-glycoprotein-mediated multidrug resistance by curcumin and vitamin D3 increases sensitivity to paclitaxel in breast cancer. Chemico-Biological Interactions. 2020;**315**(5):108865

[85] Man S, Jingwen Y, Lv P, Liu Y, Yang L, Ma L. Curcumin-enhanced antitumor effects of sorafenib via regulating the metabolism and tumor microenvironment. Food & Function. 2020;**11**:6422-6432

[86] Sahdeo Prasad PS, Chatterjee B, Chaudhary AA, Lall R, Srivastava AK. Complexity of tumor microenvironment: Therapeutic role of curcumin and its metabolites. Nutrition and Cancer. 2023;**75**(1):1-13

[87] Greil R et al. A phase 1 dose-escalation study on the safety, tolerability and activity of liposomal curcumin (Lipocurc™) in patients with locally advanced or metastatic cancer. Cancer Chemotherapy and Pharmacology. 2018;**82**(4):695-706

[88] Carroll RE et al. Phase IIa clinical trial of curcumin for the prevention of colorectal neoplasia. Cancer Prevention Research (Philadelphia, Pa.). 2011;**4**(3):354-364

[89] Kuriakose MA et al. A randomized double-blind placebo-controlled phase IIB trial of curcumin in oral leukoplakia. Cancer Prevention Research (Philadelphia, Pa.). 2016;**9**(8):683-691

[90] Toden S et al. Curcumin mediates chemosensitization to 5-fluorouracil through miRNA-induced suppression of epithelial-to-mesenchymal transition in chemoresistant colorectal cancer. Carcinogenesis. 2015;**36**(3):355-367

[91] Zhou Q et al. Curcumin improves the tumoricidal effect of mitomycin C by suppressing ABCG2 expression in stem cell-like breast cancer cells. PLoS One. 2015;**10**(8):e0136694

[92] Tabanelli R, Brogi S, Calderone V. Improving curcumin bioavailability: Current strategies and future perspectives. Pharmaceutics. 2021;**13**(10):1715

[93] Hegde M et al. Curcumin formulations for better bioavailability: What we learned from clinical trials thus far? ACS Omega. 2023;**8**(12):10713-10746

[94] Zinat Heidari MD, Boozari M, Jamialahmadi T, Sahebkar A. Curcumin supplementation in pediatric patients: A systematic review of current clinical evidence. Phytotherapy Research. 2021;**36**(4):1442-1458

[95] Hao M et al. Pharmacological mechanisms and clinical applications of curcumin: Update. Aging and Disease. 2023;**14**(3):716-749

[96] Di Meo F et al. Curcumin, gut microbiota, and neuroprotection. Nutrients. 2019;**11**(10):2426

[97] Han Z, Lu Y, Zhong Y, Xiao Y, Gao J, Zheng Z, et al. Gut microbiota mediates the effects of curcumin on enhancing Ucp1-dependent thermogenesis and improving high-fat diet-induced obesity. Food & Function. 2021;**12**(14):6558-6575

[98] Shuo Li JY, Wang Z, Liu Y, Wang B, Du M, Zou T. Curcumin alleviates high-fat diet-induced hepatic steatosis and obesity in association with modulation of gut microbiota in mice. Food Research International. 2021;**143**:110270

[99] Scazzocchio B, Minghetti L, D'Archivio M. Interaction between gut microbiota and curcumin: A new key of understanding for the health effects of curcumin. Nutrients. 2020;**12**(9):2499

[100] Saeedeh Keyvani-Ghamsari KK, Gul A. Curcumin effect on cancer cells' multidrug resistance: An update. Phytotherapy Research. 2020;**34**(10):2534-2556

Chapter 6

Nanocurcumin Formulations for Immunotherapy of Cancer

Sitabja Mukherjee and Santosh K. Kar

Abstract

American Cancer Society reported in April 2024 that about 20 million new cancer cases were diagnosed worldwide in 2020, and there were 9.7 million deaths. By 2050, this number will increase to 35 million due to population growth, aging, and lifestyle changes, with a proportionate increase in number of deaths. Therefore, there is an urgent need to reduce death by making facilities for early detection and treatment of cancer patients available at an affordable cost. Using surgery, chemo and radiation therapy doctors have been treating cancer patients till now. But after understanding how the immune system controls tumors, Immunotherapy using specific checkpoint inhibitors like anti-CTLA4 or PD-1 antibodies to block the progression of tumors and cellular therapy like CAR T-cell therapy in which T cells isolated from the patient's blood were altered by expressing *chimeric antigen receptors* (CAR) on their surfaces which when injected back into the donor can kill the cancer cells effectively more therapeutic options became available. But they cannot be used for all types of cancers, are donor-specific, and are very expensive. We will have to develop many more mono-specific immunotherapies for all types of cancer and combine them to test their effectiveness. Here, we will discuss how curcumin obtained from *Curcuma longa* plant, after being converted into bioavailable nanoformulations, can be fed orally to cancer patients to modulate the gut microbiota, which would in turn alter the immunosuppressive environment inside the tumor microbiomes and kill cancer cells more effectively with less toxicity.

Keywords: nanocurcumin, bioavailable formulations, oral administration, modulation of gut and tumor microbiome, antibody and cell-based immunotherapy, improved quality of life

1. Introduction

Treating cancer patients to save their life and reducing toxicity, which would improve the quality of their life while undergoing treatment at an early stage at an affordable cost, is the need of the hour and is the responsibility of the medical scientists. Therefore, long before the present-day therapeutic options for the treatment of cancer became available, various methods that could save life were tried. Doctors were using infection with different bacteria to cure malignancies. Among numerous such efforts was that of William B. Coley, a New York-based surgeon who used a bacterial vaccine to treat primarily inoperable sarcoma and accomplished a 1 in 10 cure rate [1]. At that time, no one knew how infection with certain bacteria helped in the regression of tumors, and patients were

IntechOpen

reluctant to use such type of treatment. But now we know that inside a tumor, the cancer cells survive by creating an immunosuppressive milieu, and when the administered bacteria alters it, the cancer cells cannot survive anymore. This has opened up a new approach for microbial therapy using many bacterial species including *Mycobacterium Bovis Bacillus Calmette-Guérin* (BCG) for cancer treatment [2]. BCG was developed in 1921s for use as a vaccine for tuberculosis, but the observation that tuberculosis patients usually had a lower incidence of cancer raised the possibility that *Mycobacterium tuberculosis* infection may confer protection against different types of cancers. Experimental evidence that immunization with BCG can protect against various types of cancers like lymphoblastoid leukemia, colon cancer, lung cancer, and melanoma emerged during the 1950s and 1960s, and now doctors treat non-muscle-invasive bladder cancer by injecting BCG directly into the bladder for its effective regression [3].

With surgical intervention already at their disposal when chemotherapy and radiotherapy became available, doctors used them for treatment and moved away from bacterial therapy. But in the recent past interest in bacterial therapies has resurfaced again [4].

With the availability of technologies for the production of monoclonal antibodies specific against tumor cell surface antigens and approval by the food and drug administration (FDA) for the use of some of them like imatinib and trastuzumab which could kill cancer cells by binding to molecules found only on cancer cell surfaces "targeted therapies" became a part of standard treatment protocol. Due to the immunogenicity of mouse monoclonal antibodies, when injected repeatedly into humans, they were humanized and used. Some antibodies were conjugated with drugs or biological toxins and when injected into patients with lymphoma, breast cancer, head and neck (HNC), and colorectal carcinomas (CRC) they could kill cancer cells more effectively [5].

While efforts to develop monoclonal antibody-based therapies were continuing many new immunotherapies were conceptualized, tested and approved during the years when the SARS-2 virus pandemic was devastating the world. One such therapy was the vaccine for prostate cancer patients [6]. This vaccine used autologous dendritic cells from the patient, which were cultured and reintroduced into the patient to induce antibody response against prostate cancer cells and prolonged patients' survival.

T cells mature in the thymus and circulate in the periphery to respond to antigens, which are presented to them by autologous antigen-presenting cells. T cells, after getting activated and performing their effector function, should not continue to circulate and create cytokine storm condition that harms the host. Therefore, T cells use molecules like CTLA4 and PD-1 expressed on their surface to act as a breakpoint, which can dampen the immune response.

Tumors present in the tissue take advantage of this dampening process to survive and grow [7]. Thus, an idea emerged that if antibodies to these cell surface molecules, which are called immune checkpoint inhibitors (ICIs)would be prepared and injected into cancer patients, they may lift the inhibition and allow the T cells to proliferate and kill the tumor and act as a therapy for cancer.

After immune checkpoint inhibitors (ICIs) were developed and were shown to work in mouse models, it was approved for use to treat cancer patients. They became the fourth arm of cancer therapy. Ipilimumaban anti-CTLA4 antibody was the first checkpoint inhibitor to be used for the treatment of stage IV melanoma patients in melanoma clinical trials and showed great potential. Many patients were cured, while a large number of them showed toxicity and experienced relapse. Better results with much less toxicity were observed when antibodies like nivolumab and pembrolizumab against another checkpoint inhibitor PD-1 were used for therapy [8]. For this magnificent contribution, the Nobel Prize for Physiology or Medicine was awarded to Profs. James P Allison from the USA and Tasuku Honjo from Japan in the year 2018.

After decades of research and a better understanding of our immune system, therapies that can use patient's own T cells were developed. For this, T cells from the patient were isolated and modified in the laboratory to express receptors that can recognize specific molecules on the cancer cell surfaces of the donor. When such cells were injected back, they could kill the cancer cells in the patient using cytotoxic mechanisms [9].

With success achieved by using these ICIs and CAR T cells as monotherapies for cancer, numerous immunotherapies were developed and tested alone or in combination for efficacy.

For example, when CAR T cells were used in combination with anti-PD1 antibody in lymphoma patients it showed better cytotoxicity [10]. Clinical studies have shown that persons with lower NK cell cytotoxicity are more prone to get cancer. Since NK cells are not regulated by MHC antigens, use will not be restricted only to autologous conditions, and off-the-self manufacturing will be an advantage. Infusion of NK cells with antibodies and cytokines has already been demonstrated, and soon, NK cell therapy will be available for patient use [11]. Macrophages play an important role in maintaining the tumor microenvironment and have a role in the immunological orchestra, such as angiogenesis, extracellular matrix remodeling, and metastasis, which plays out for the survival of the cancer cells inside the tumor. When activated macrophages are introduced they can increase phagocytosis of cancer cells and killing by cytotoxic mechanisms. Therefore, the use of activated macrophages will be very helpful for cancer therapy [12]. There have been numerous reports about the feasibility of DC-based immunotherapies for cancer patients, but the clinical benefits are not as much as anticipated. Therefore more research needs to be done to understand the future of DC therapy for tumor control [13]. Tumors create enormously complex microenvironments for their survival and proliferation in the tissue. Some of the cells which play a dominant role are fibroblasts and stromal cells [14]. When research establishes their usefulness for cellular therapy and they will become available for use, they can be tested individually or in combination with other monotherapy for efficacy [14, 15]. Curcumin is very insoluble in water and under physiologic conditions, can be degraded rapidly into different components and can be metabolized by enzymes into more soluble derivatives [16]. When taken orally, curcumin comes in direct contact with trillions of microbiota present in the gut and changes their composition and function. For centuries, turmeric has been used in Indian traditional system as an antibacterial, anti-inflammatory, and wound-healing agent. In recent times it has been shown to improve the metabolic health of humans by promoting the secretion of certain metabolites and reducing the production of lipopolysaccharide (LPS) by bacteria, which induces inflammation. In order to make curcumin effective against the tumor microbiome and reduce the progression of the tumor, we will have to study it further.

The coming decade may see the removal of the obstacles that exist today, and with the identification of new targets and biomarkers, cancer immune therapy may become an effective and affordable option for the treatment of certain cancer types.

2. The Curcuma longa plant: Natural curcumin and making it bioavailable for use

Curcuma longa linn is the plant from whose rhisome curcumin is isolated. It belongs to the Zingiberaceae family and grows in tropical climates requiring significant rainfall. It does not have a seed and is propagated from the rhizome. The rhizome, after boiling in water, drying, and then making it into powder, is used as turmeric to spice up our curries. In the Indian traditional system of medicine, it has been used for centuries as an antibacterial agent, a wound healer, and for reducing pain without knowing which component of it is responsible for these medicinal properties. When Vogel and Pelletier isolated the molecule for the first time in pure form, research to determine its structure and function was started [16].

Milobedzka and Lampe identified the chemical structure of this molecule in 1910 and named it as curcumin [17]. The same group synthesized it in the laboratory in 1913 [18]. Finally, Srinivasan separated and quantified the components of curcumin by chromatography and showed that it is a mixture of three molecules, namely curcumin, demethoxycurcumin, and bis-demethoxycurcumin [19].

The rhizome of the *Curcuma longa* plant contains besides the *curcumin* (curcumin I), which is the principal *curcuminoid*, three other *curcuminoids*, namely *demethoxy-curcumin* (curcumin II), *bisdemethoxycurcumin* (curcumin III), and the recently identified cyclocurcumin in the following approximate proportions namely 75–80% curcumin, 15–20% demethoxycurcumin, 3–5% bisdemethoxycurcumin and trace amount of cyclocurcumin [20]. Curcumin has two electron-rich aromatic rings containing o-methoxy phenolic groups at either end of the molecule, which are connected by an α,β-unsaturated β-diketone seven-member chain, which allows it to exhibit keto-enol tautomerism. In the enol form, curcumin has to be a planar molecule to allow the π electron cloud from the aromatic rings to spread all over the molecule. It is a hydrophobic molecule with a logP value of ~3.0 and is almost insoluble in water but dissolves in solvents like methanol, acetone, ethyl alcohol, etc. Curcumin absorbs in the visible range of 410–430 nm and in the UV range of 265 nm.

Although curcumin is safe and well-tolerated even at high doses, its poor bioavailability has limited its pharmaceutical use. Oral doses result in minimal serum concentrations due to poor absorption, rapid metabolism, and elimination. For instance, even a 2 g/kg oral dose in rats yields peak serum levels of only ~1.35 μg/mL [21]. Similarly, human trials with oral doses up to 3.6 g showed extremely low systemic levels [22–25]. To overcome these challenges, modern strategies like nanoformulations have been developed. These include nanoparticles, liposomes, and nanoemulsions made from materials such as PLGA, chitosan, silk fibroin, and NIPAAM [26–30]. These delivery systems, each involving distinct preparation processes, aim to improve curcumin's solubility, protect it from degradation, and enable targeted drug release in diseased tissues, enhancing therapeutic efficacy while reducing side effects.

Nanoprecipitation dissolves curcumin in a solvent and then precipitates it into nanoparticles in an aqueous phase [31]. Emulsification-solvent evaporation forms an emulsion of curcumin in an organic solvent, which is then evaporated to yield nanoparticles [32]. Liposomal encapsulation traps curcumin within phospholipid vesicles, while SLNs embed it in a solid lipid matrix [33, 34]. Polymeric nanoparticles use biodegradable polymers like PLGA or chitosan for encapsulation [35, 36]. Nanoemulsions, micelles, and SMEDDS create stable dispersions in aqueous systems [37–40]. Emerging methods include supercritical fluid processing, electrospinning, and dendrimer-based formulations for targeted delivery [41–43]. Nanocurcumin exhibits higher plasma concentrations compared to conventional curcumin formulations. This improvement is attributed to the reduced particle size, which enhances cellular uptake and transcellular transport, thereby increasing the absorption of curcumin into the bloodstream from the gut (**Figure 1**). Nanocurcumin, due to its larger surface area, has greater interaction with serum albumin and other serum

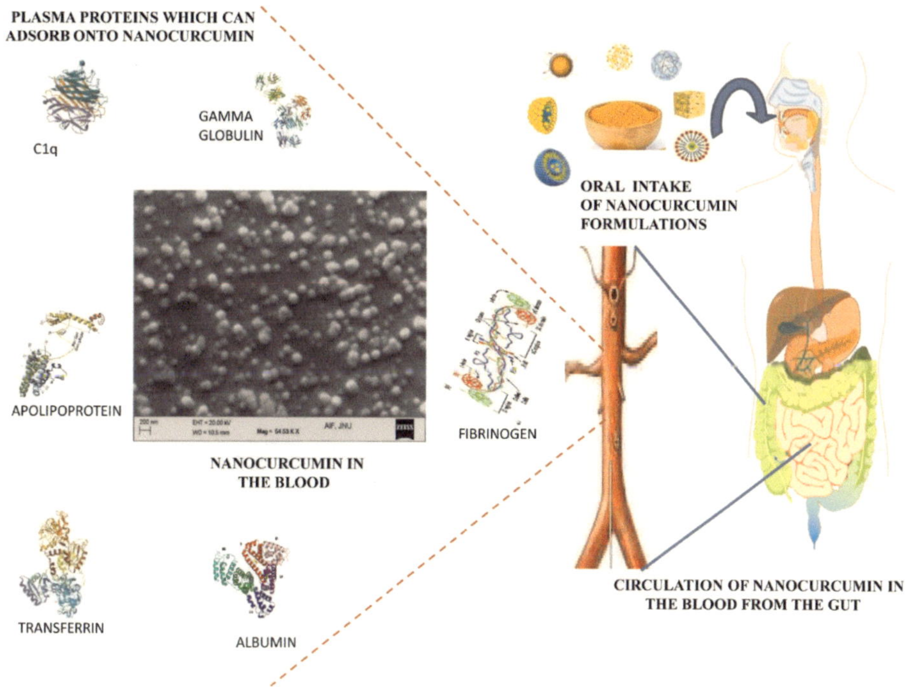

Figure 1.
Oral intake of formulations containing nanocurcumin results in the nanoparticles reaching the gut and circulating in the blood via *the portal vein. Due to an increase in the surface area of the nanoparticles and affinity to proteins like albumin, gamma globulin, etc., present in the blood, the nanoparticles get coated with these proteins, become resistant to enzymatic conversion, and circulate for longer periods in the tissue and exhibit anticancer activity.*

proteins, which shields it from rapid hepatic metabolism, thereby allowing it to circulate for a prolonged period and modulate key oncogenic pathways by both direct and indirect interactions. Both the direct and indirect targets encompass a broad spectrum of functionally significant molecules, including several transcription factors, enzymes, protein kinases, inflammatory mediators, growth factors, receptors, and drug-resistance proteins. Additionally, many adhesion molecules, chemokines, and their receptors, cell-cycle regulators, and proteins governing cell survival and apoptosis also fall into these categories. By modulating these components, curcumin can influence numerous cellular processes such as proliferation, differentiation, inflammation, immune response, and cell death—processes that are often dysregulated in cancer. A detailed list of important targets that curcumin can influence is given in **Table 1.**

3. Evaluating the efficacy of Nanocurcumin in cancer therapy: Insights from clinical trials

A growing body of clinical evidence has explored the therapeutic potential of nanocurcumin in mitigating the adverse effects of cancer therapies and enhancing treatment outcomes across various malignancies. In the context of cisplatin-induced nephrotoxicity, two randomized clinical trials yielded mixed findings. One study involving 82 patients demonstrated that nanocurcumin significantly improved blood urea nitrogen (BUN) and glomerular filtration rate (GFR), indicating a protective effect

Category	Targets	Effect
Transcription factors	Activating transcription factor-3	Downregulation
	Activator protein-1	Downregulation
	β-Catenin	Downregulation
	CREB-binding protein	Downregulation
	C/EBP homologous protein	Downregulation
	Electrophile response element	Upregulation
	Early growth response gene-1	Downregulation
	Hypoxia-inducible factor-1α	Downregulation
	Nuclear factor κ-B	Downregulation
	Notch-1	Downregulation
	NFE2-related factor	Upregulation
	p53	Upregulation
	Peroxisome-proliferator-activated receptor-γ	Upregulation
	Specificity protein-1	Downregulation
	STAT-1	Downregulation
	STAT-3	Downregulation
	STAT-4	Downregulation
	STAT-5	Downregulation
	Wilms' tumor gene 1	Downregulation
Inflammatory mediators	C-reactive protein	Downregulation
	Interleukin 1β	Downregulation
	Interleukin 2	Downregulation
	Interleukin 5	Downregulation
	Interleukin 6	Downregulation
	Interleukin 8	Downregulation
	Interleukin 12	Downregulation
	Interleukin 18	Downregulation
	Interferon γ	Downregulation
	Inducible nitric oxide synthase	Downregulation
	5-Lipoxygenase	Downregulation
	Monocyte chemoattractant protein	Downregulation
	Migration inhibition protein	Downregulation
	Macrophage inflammatory protein-1α	Downregulation
	Prostate-specific antigen	Downregulation
Growth Factors	Connective tissue growth factor	Downregulation
	Epidermal growth factor	Downregulation
	Fibroblast growth factor	Downregulation
	HER2	Downregulation

Category	Targets	Effect
	Hepatocyte growth factor	Downregulation
	Platelet-derived growth factor	Downregulation
	Tissue factor Downregulation Transforming growth factor-β1 Downregulation	
	Chemokine ligand 1 ↓	Downregulation
	Chemokine ligand 2 ↓	Downregulation
Chemokines, chemokine receptors and cell adhesion molecules	Chemokine receptors 4 ↓	Downregulation
	Intracellular adhesion molecule-1	Downregulation
	Endothelial leukocyte adhesion molecule-1	Downregulation
	Vascular cell adhesion molecule-1	Downregulation
Enzymes and Protein kinases	Acetylcholinesterase	Downregulation
	Aldose reductase	Downregulation
	Arylamine N-acetyltransferases-1	Downregulation
	Beta-site APP-cleaving enzyme-1	Downregulation
	CD13	Downregulation
	DNA polymerase I	Downregulation
	DNA topoisomerase-II	Downregulation
	GTPase (microtubule assembly)	Downregulation
	Glutathione reductase	Downregulation
	Glutathione-peroxidase	Downregulation
	Glutathione S transferase	Upregulation
	Hemeoxygenase 1	Upregulation
	Ca^{2+}-dependent ATPase	Downregulation
	Inosine monophosphate dehydrogenase	Downregulation
	17β-HSD3	Downregulation
	Ornithine decarboxylase	Downregulation
	Monoamine oxidase	Downregulation
	NADP(H):quinoneoxidoreductase 1	Downregulation
	Phospholipase D	Downregulation
	Thioredoxin reductase 1	Downregulation
	Telomerase	Downregulation
	Ubiquitin isopeptidases	Downregulation
	Ca^{2+}, phospholipid-dependent protein kinase C	Downregulation
	c-jun N-terminal kinase	Downregulation
	cAMP-dependent protein kinase	Downregulation
	CSN-associated kinase	Downregulation
	CSN-associated kinase	Downregulation

Category	Targets	Effect
EGF receptor kinase	Downregulation	
	Extracellular receptor kinase	Downregulation
	Focal adhesion kinase	Downregulation
	IL-1 receptor-associated kinase	Downregulation
	IκB kinase	Downregulation
	Janus kinase	Downregulation
	Mitogen-activated protein kinase	Downregulation
	pp60c-src tyrosine kinase	Downregulation
	Phosphorylase kinase	Downregulation
	Protein kinase A	Downregulation
	PI3K-Akt	Downregulation
	Protamine kinase	Downregulation
Chemokines, chemokine receptors and cell adhesion molecules	Chemokine receptors 4 ↓	Downregulation
	Intracellular adhesion molecule-1	Downregulation
	Endothelial leukocyte adhesion molecule-1	Downregulation
	Vascular cell adhesion molecule-1	Downregulation
Enzymes and Protein kinases	Acetylcholinesterase	Downregulation
	Aldose reductase	Downregulation
	Arylamine N-acetyltransferases-1	Downregulation
	Beta-site APP-cleaving enzyme-1	Downregulation
	CD13	Downregulation
	DNA polymerase I	Downregulation
	DNA topoisomerase-II	Downregulation
	GTPase (microtubule assembly)	Downregulation
	Glutathione reductase	Downregulation
	Glutathione-peroxidase	Downregulation
	Glutathione S-transferase	Upregulation
	Hemeoxygenase 1	Upregulation
	Ca^{2+}-dependent ATPase	Downregulation
	Inosine monophosphate dehydrogenase	Downregulation
	17β-HSD3	Downregulation
	Ornithine decarboxylase	Downregulation
	Monoamine oxidase	Downregulation
	NADP(H):quinoneoxidoreductase 1	Downregulation
	Phospholipase D	Downregulation
	Thioredoxin reductase 1	Downregulation
	Telomerase	Downregulation
	Ubiquitin isopeptidases	Downregulation

Category	Targets	Effect
	Ca^{2+}, phospholipid-dependent protein kinase C	Downregulation
	c-jun N-terminal kinase	Downregulation
	cAMP-dependent protein kinase	Downregulation
	CSN-associated kinase	Downregulation
	CSN-associated kinase	Downregulation
	EGF receptor kinase	Downregulation
	Extracellular receptor kinase	Downregulation
	Focal adhesion kinase	Downregulation
	IL-1 receptor-associated kinase	Downregulation
	IκB kinase	Downregulation
	Janus kinase	Downregulation
	Mitogen-activated protein kinase	Downregulation
	pp60c-src tyrosine kinase	Downregulation
	Phosphorylase kinase	Downregulation
	Protein kinase A	Downregulation
	PI3K-Akt	Downregulation
	Protamine kinase	Downregulation
Cell-cycle regulatory proteins and invasion biomarkers	Cyclin D1	Downregulation
	Cyclin E	Downregulation
	c-Myc	Downregulation
	p21	Downregulation
	Matrix metalloproteinase-9	Downregulation
	Urokinase-type plasminogen activator	Downregulation
	Vascular endothelial growth factor	Downregulation
Receptors	Androgen receptor	Downregulation
	Aryl hydrocarbon receptor	Downregulation
	Death receptor-5	Downregulation
	EGF receptor	Downregulation
	Endothelial protein C-receptor	Downregulation
	Estrogen receptor-α	Downregulation
	Fas	Upregulation
	Histamine 2-receptor	Downregulation
	Interleukin 8-receptor	Downregulation
	Inositol 1,4,5-triphosphate receptor	Downregulation
	Integrin receptor	Downregulation
	Low-density lipoprotein-receptor	Upregulation
	Transferrin receptor 1	Downregulation

Category	Targets	Effect
Others	cAMP response element binding protein	Downregulation
	DNA fragmentation factor 40-kDa subunit	Downregulation
	Fibrinogen	Downregulation
	Ferritin H and L	Downregulation
	Heat-shock protein 70	Upregulation
	Multi-drug resistance protein-1	Downregulation
	Multi-drug resistance protein-2	Downregulation

Table 1.
List of key transcription factors, enzymes, protein kinases, inflammatory mediators, growth factors, receptors, chemokines, adhesion molecules, cell-cycle regulators, and proteins that are modulated by interaction with curcumin.

against tubular toxicity, although changes in other renal markers were not statistically significant [44]. Conversely, another smaller trial involving 30 patients reported no significant difference in renal function or acute kidney injury incidence between treatment and placebo groups, suggesting limited nephroprotection at the administered dosage [45]. In addressing radiation-induced skin reactions (RISRs) among breast cancer patients, a triple-blind, placebo-controlled trial found that daily administration of nanocurcumin during radiotherapy led to a statistically significant reduction in RISR severity by the seventh week and decreased pain scores, although early-phase differences were not observed [46]. Similarly, a double-blind study evaluating nanocurcumin as an adjunct therapy in muscle-invasive bladder cancer indicated a higher complete response rate in the treatment group compared to placebo (50% vs. 30.8%) [47]. In patients undergoing radiotherapy for prostate cancer, nanocurcumin supplementation was well-tolerated but failed to demonstrate significant reductions in radiation-induced proctitis, cystitis, or hematologic toxicity [48]. A trial examining nanocurcumin's cardioprotective role during doxorubicin-based chemotherapy in breast cancer patients revealed that left ventricular function remained stable in the nanocurcumin group, in contrast to significant deterioration in the placebo group, indicating a potential benefit in preserving cardiac function [49]. Finally, in head and neck cancer patients, a randomized trial comparing a 0.1% nanocurcumin-based mouthwash to 0.15% benzydamine demonstrated that curcumin significantly delayed the onset of radiation-induced oral mucositis (RIOM) by nearly 2 weeks [50]. Collectively, these findings highlight nanocurcumin's potential in reducing the severity and onset of treatment-related toxicities and possibly improving therapeutic response.

4. The gut microbiome in the context of Nanocurcumin: But now also the influence on the tumor microbiome?

The human gut contains around 40 trillion microorganisms that play vital roles in digestion, immunity, and disease susceptibility, including cancer. Recent research has uncovered the gut-tumor microbiome axis, where both gut and tumor-resident microbes significantly influence cancer development and treatment response. A large-scale study analyzing over 1500 tumor samples from seven cancer types detected specific bacterial communities within tumors, highlighting the presence of a distinct intratumoral microbiome [51]. Disruptions in microbial balance can produce carcinogenic metabolites, promote inflammation, and impair treatment outcomes [52]. One example is *Fusobacterium nucleatum*, which promotes colorectal cancer by activating β-catenin signaling, suppressing natural killer cell function, and contributing to chemotherapy resistance.

Curcumin has emerged as a potential modulator of the gut microbiota, which supports regulatory T-cell balance, modulates dendritic cell activity, and inhibits pathways like indoleamine 2,3-dioxygenase (IDO) that suppress immune responses [53]. These actions enhance its potential synergy with immune checkpoint inhibitors. Gut microbiota composition has been shown to influence immunotherapy outcomes, with specific bacteria like *Faecalibacterium prausnitzii* and *Akkermansia muciniphila* linked to better responses [54, 55].

Nanocurcumin has been shown to reach tumor tissues more effectively than its native counterpart and interact with gut microbes, increasing beneficial species like *Lactobacillus*, *Bifidobacterium*, and *Akkermansia*, while reducing harmful taxa such as Prevotellaceae and Enterobacteriaceae (**Figure 2**). These properties make nanocurcumin particularly suited for modulating both gut and tumor-associated microbiota for therapeutic purposes. Building on the foundations of gut microbial modulation, emerging research has shifted attention toward the tumor microbiome—microbial communities that reside within tumor tissues themselves [56]. This compartment harbors unique bacterial populations distinct from those in surrounding healthy tissues, and their functional relevance is becoming increasingly apparent.

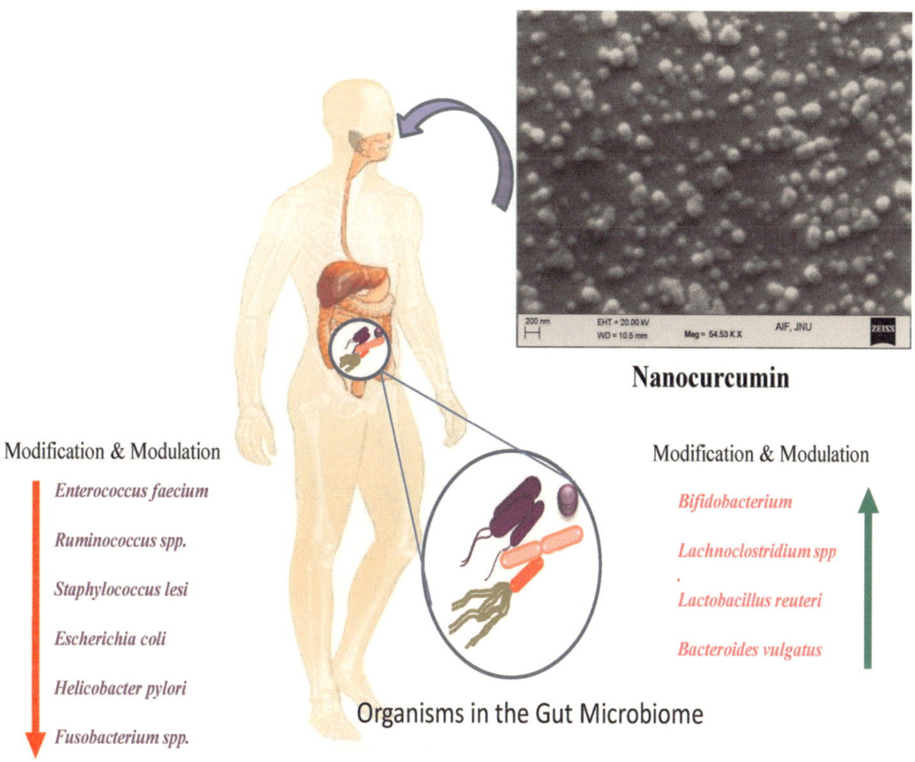

Figure 2.
On oral delivery, nanocurcumin reaches the gut and interacts with the gut microbiota, modulating their composition and metabolism. Some microbiota get upregulated and secrete metabolites, which affect cancer cells in the tumor microbiome.

Recent technologies have enabled the identification of tumor-associated microbial populations, demonstrating that the diversity of intratumoral microbiota varies across different types of cancer. Lung tumors harbor *Modestobacter*, *Blastomyces*, and *Klebsiella*, while liver cancer tissues frequently contain hepatitis B and C viruses, *Helicobacter pylori*, and *Gammaproteobacteria*. Colorectal cancer is strongly associated with *Fusobacterium nucleatum* and enterotoxigenic *Bacteroides fragilis*, which promote inflammation and immune evasion. Gastric cancer microbiota is dominated by *H. pylori*, Epstein–Barr virus, and lactobacilli, influencing carcinogenesis through immune modulation and epigenetic alterations. Breast cancer exhibits high bacterial diversity, including *Pseudomonas*, *Proteus*, and *Methylobacterium radiotolerans*, with potential implications for tumor progression. Pancreatic cancer microbiota is enriched with *Proteobacteria*, *Pseudomonas*, and *Malassezia*, while oral cancer features pathogenic species, such as *F. nucleatum*, *P. gingivalis*, and *Streptococcus anginosus*, which contribute to carcinogenesis through DNA damage and inflammatory pathways. Notably, microbial compositions also correlate with tumor histological subtypes, stages, and genetic mutations. These tumor-resident microbes can modulate oncogenic pathways, alter local immune landscapes, and influence the efficacy of immune checkpoint blockade therapies [57]. Given this context, modulating the tumor microbiome represents a novel avenue for improving cancer treatment outcomes, especially in immunotherapy. Curcumin, particularly in its nanoformulated form, offers a novel strategy to modulate the diversity of these intratumoral microbial ecosystems present in different types of cancers (**Figure 3**). Further studies should

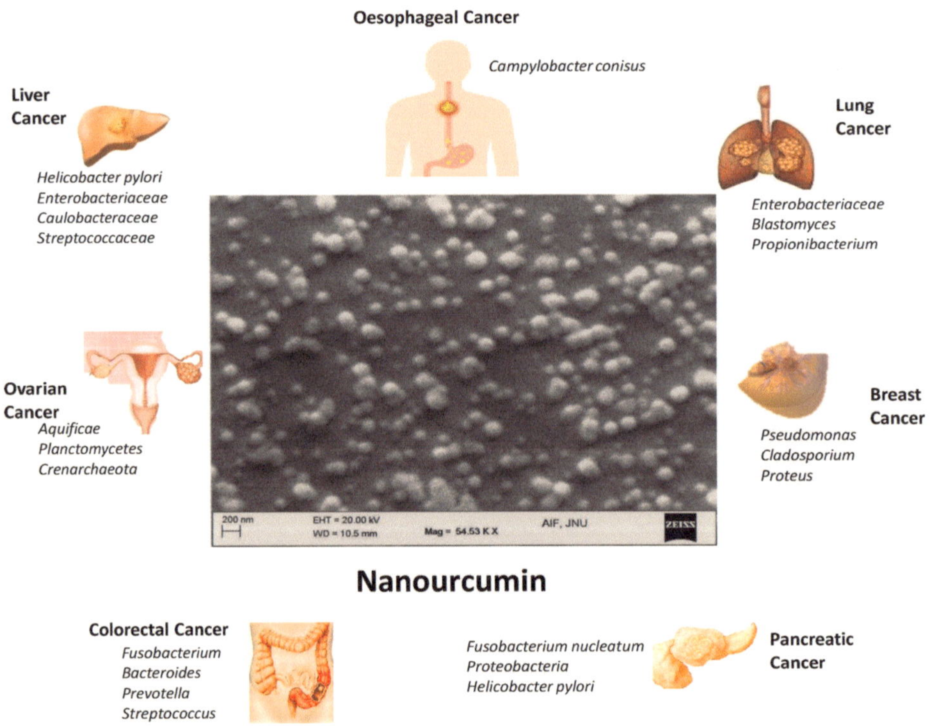

Figure 3.
Seven different tumor microbiomes with different microbiota have been identified. Curcumin nanoparticles and the metabolites secreted by gut microbiome after interacting with curcumin therefore will have different effect on them.

explore how nanocurcumin can bridge gut and tumor microbiota modulation with improved immune responses and augmented cancer treatment efficacy.

5. Discussion

Cancer remains a formidable therapeutic challenge with no universally effective treatment strategy. Among emerging modalities, immunotherapy and curcumin-based interventions have demonstrated significant potential but are constrained by critical limitations.

Immunotherapy, which augments the host immune response against tumor cells, has achieved notable success in hematologic malignancies. However, its efficacy in solid tumors is limited due to tumor heterogeneity, immune resistance, and the immunosuppressive tumor microenvironment (TME). Within the TME, regulatory T cells, tumor-associated macrophages, and myeloid-derived suppressor cells secrete inhibitory cytokines such as TGF-β and IL-10, suppressing effector immune functions [58]. Additionally, approaches like (CAR) T-cell therapy faces challenges in solid tumors, including poor infiltration, antigen-driven exhaustion, and structural barriers such as abnormal vasculature and extracellular matrix density. Continued investigation into the mechanisms underlying immune evasion, therapeutic resistance, and tumor complexity is essential to enhancing the clinical utility of these interventions. The development of next-generation CAR T cells aims to address these challenges by incorporating co-stimulatory signals, cytokine secretion mechanisms, and enhanced trafficking capabilities. Despite its efficacy in certain settings, immunotherapy is associated with severe adverse effects that limit its application. One of the most significant toxicities is cytokine storm involving overproduction of cytokines such as IL-1, IL-6, and IFN-γ, resulting in multi-organ failure, necessitating intensive medical management.

Neurotoxicity is another concern, particularly in CAR T-cell therapy, where immune infiltration into the central nervous system can lead to encephalopathy, seizures, and cognitive impairment [59]. These toxicities highlight the need for improving therapeutic outcomes and minimizing harm.

While immunotherapy is there to stay natural compounds such as curcumin have garnered attention for their potential as chemopreventive and adjunctive therapies for cancer.

Curcumin has been extensively studied for its anticancer potential due to its ability to disrupt key cancer hallmarks, including resistance to apoptosis, angiogenesis, uncontrolled cell proliferation, invasion, metastasis, and resistance to growth-regulating signals. It exerts anticancer effects through multiple pathways, including the inhibition of NF-κB, modulation of MAPK and JNK signaling, and downregulation of pro-inflammatory cytokines. Beyond its role in influencing T-cell activity, curcumin has been found to enhance the cytotoxic capabilities of tumor-suppressed effector T cells. Studies have demonstrated that curcumin significantly increases CD86 expression on dendritic cells while reducing the effector T-cell-mediated secretion of pro-inflammatory cytokines [60]. Adoptive T-cell therapy, a rapidly growing field in cancer immunotherapy, involves reinfusing a patient's own expanded effector T cells to increase the number of tumor-fighting immune cells. However, the immunosuppressive nature of the tumor microenvironment often limits the long-term success of this approach. Interestingly, the combination of adoptive T-cell therapy with curcumin has shown promising results. In a mouse model of E.G7 T lymphoma, curcumin was found to enhance CD8+ T-cell infiltration into tumors following adoptive cell transfer, as well as increase the production of interferons (IFN) by CD8+ T cells [60]. This combination therapy demonstrated greater efficacy in suppressing tumor growth compared to T-cell therapy alone. These findings suggest that integrating curcumin into immunotherapeutic strategies may provide new opportunities for cancer treatment and management and could significantly improve treatment outcomes [61].

Chronic pain is a significant clinical challenge in oncology, often arising due to tumor progression, inflammatory responses, nerve compression, and adverse effects of chemotherapy, radiotherapy, and surgery. The complex pathophysiology of cancer pain involves multiple molecular and cellular mechanisms, including the activation of inflammatory pathways, oxidative stress, and neuroimmune interactions. Addressing this multifaceted nature of pain requires therapeutic agents capable of modulating these underlying processes. Curcumin's analgesic effects are attributed to its ability to downregulate pro-inflammatory cytokines such as TNF-α, IL-6, and IL-1β, inhibit the NF-κB signaling pathway, and modulate the activity of COX-2 and iNOS, which are key mediators of inflammation and pain sensitization. A study assessing the efficacy of nanocurcumin and curcumin in chronic pain management analyzed data from 59 studies, including 29 preclinical and 30 clinical investigations [62]. Preclinical studies demonstrated a significant analgesic effect of curcumin, with both oral and intraperitoneal administration yielding statistically significant pain reduction, while subcutaneous administration showed no measurable impact. The therapeutic efficacy was most pronounced within the 100–250 mg dosage range, with diminishing benefits at higher doses, suggesting a dose-dependent response within an optimal therapeutic window. Clinical studies further corroborated these findings, indicating that nanocurcumin exhibited a superior analgesic effect in comparison to placebo [62]. Enhanced bioavailability formulations of curcumin also demonstrated greater efficacy in pain reduction compared to conventional curcumin extracts [62]. Notably, curcumin administration did not interfere with the analgesic effects of NSAIDs when used in combination, is suggestive of its application as a potential adjunct therapy to standard regimens for the effective management of pain. This is of particular importance in cancer patients, as long-term NSAID use is often limited by gastrointestinal and renal side effects, whereas curcumin has demonstrated a favorable safety profile. Beyond direct analgesic effects, curcumin has been shown to exert neuroprotective and neuromodulatory actions by inhibiting microglial activation and suppressing central sensitization mechanisms that contribute to neuropathic pain, a common complication in cancer patients undergoing chemotherapy. Additionally, curcumin's immunomodulatory properties, including its ability to regulate T-cell responses and reduce chronic inflammation, may further contribute to its analgesic potential in the tumor microenvironment. These findings underscore the potential of curcumin and its nanoformulations as promising therapeutic agents for alleviating cancer-related pain and treatment-induced toxicities, contributing to an improved quality of life for patients. However, while preclinical and early-phase clinical studies demonstrate encouraging results, additional randomized controlled trials on a larger scale are required to confirm and validate the existent results, optimize dosing strategies, and establish standardized treatment protocols for integration into oncological pain management.

One of the primary challenges associated with curcumin therapy is the inconsistency in curcumin preparations. Early strategies to enhance curcumin's bioavailability centered on using natural adjuvants such as turmeric oil, fibers (e.g., BCM-95 and

Cureit), or turmeric oleoresin (Curcugen) to stabilize curcumin in its active form [63]. Another method involved co-administering curcumin with piperine (as in the C3 complex), which inhibits key metabolic enzymes like cytochrome P450 and UDP-glucuronyltransferase. This slows down curcumin's breakdown and prolongs its systemic presence, thereby increasing its therapeutic potential. Second-generation formulations aimed to boost solubility and absorption using delivery systems such as phospholipid complexes, lipid carriers, polysorbates, and nanoparticle technologies. Examples include BioCurc, Theracurmin, Meriva, and Nanocurcumin. Although these approaches increased plasma curcuminoid levels, most of the curcumin converted into inactive metabolites like glucuronides and sulfates. Due to their poor tissue penetration and rapid excretion. To overcome these issues, third-generation formulations were developed to deliver free, unconjugated curcumin with higher cellular uptake and membrane permeability without artificial additives [63]. The different curcumin formulations that have been used in human clinical studies have been listed in **Table 2** [63]. The term "curcumin" therefore, is often used interchangeably to describe the various formulations, including turmeric extracts, curcuminoid-enriched compounds, and purified curcumin. This lack of standardization complicates research findings, as different studies may evaluate products with varying compositions and potencies. Furthermore, attributing biological activity solely to curcumin within complex turmeric preparations raises concerns about the reproducibility and generalizability of results. Curcumin's poor bioavailability is another significant limitation that is often brought up in different studies. When taken orally, curcumin undergoes rapid metabolism and extensive first-pass clearance, resulting in low systemic concentrations. While bioavailable formulations have been developed to enhance absorption, their efficacy compared to standard curcumin remains uncertain due to a lack of rigorous comparative studies. Some evidence suggests that even unmodified curcumin may exert therapeutic effects in localized settings, such as gastrointestinal cancers, where direct tissue exposure occurs. A critical issue affecting curcumin research is the inconsistency in clinical trial design. Although randomized controlled trials investigating curcumin's effects are increasing, many are small-scale Phase II studies with substantial variability in dosing regimens, treatment duration, and proprietary formulations. Only a fraction of these trials incorporate molecular biomarkers to assess efficacy, leading to a disconnect between preclinical findings and clinical outcomes. Without standardization, it becomes a challenge to draw definitive conclusions about curcumin's role in cancer therapy and prevention. The pleiotropic nature of curcumin, while theoretically beneficial, poses additional challenges in clinical translation. Unlike targeted therapies that act on specific molecular pathways, curcumin influences multiple signaling cascades, making it difficult to pinpoint its precise mechanism of action. This broad activity complicates efforts to optimize dosing, identify predictive biomarkers, and tailor treatment to specific patient populations. Furthermore, the lack of large-scale trials evaluating curcumin's role in cancer prevention limits its potential integration into clinical practice. While some studies suggest that curcumin may reduce cancer risk in inflammatory conditions such as oral leukoplakia, ulcerative colitis, and Crohn's disease, the small sample sizes and lack of standardization prevent definitive conclusions from being drawn. Debate continues over whether bioavailable formulations of curcumin are necessary for cancer prevention and treatment. Some researchers argue that systemic absorption is essential for curcumin's therapeutic effects, while others suggest that localized activity may be sufficient for certain malignancies. It is important to note that although curcumin is known to interact with a wide range of enzymes and molecular targets, these interactions are

Curcumin formulations	Condition	Number of patients	Duration	Dosage
BCM 95	Multiple myeloma	33	28 days	8 g/day
	Multiple sclerosis	80	24 months	1 g/day
	NAFLD	50	12 weeks	1.5 g/day
	Prediabetes	84	90 days	500 mg/day
Curcumin C3 complex	MetS	117	8 weeks	1 g/day +10 mg/day
	NAFLD	70	12 weeks	500 mg/day +5 mg/day
	NAFLD	55	8 weeks	500 mg/day +5 mg/day
	NAFLD	55	8 weeks	500 mg/day +50
	NAFLD			mg/day
		102	8 weeks	1 g/day
		102	8 weeks	1 g/day
		36	8 weeks	1.5 g/day
		58	8 weeks	250 mg/day
		65	8 weeks	250 mg/day
		54	8 weeks	250 mg/day
	Osteoarthritis	50	12 weeks	1 g/day
		100	8 months	1 g/day
	Pancreatic cancer	44	until death	2 g/day 28 days cycle
	Prostatic hyperplasia	61	24 weeks	1 g/day
	Psoriasis	63	12 weeks	2 g/day
	Risk of T2D	29	12 weeks	1 g/day
Nanocurcumin (curcumin nanomicelle from Exir Nano Sina company)	Amyotrophic lateral sclerosis	54	12 months	80 mg/day
	Bladder cancer	26	4 weeks	160 mg/day
	Oral mucositis	50	7 weeks	160 mg/day
	Prostate cancer	64	3 days before radiotherapy (RT) and during RT	120 mg/day
	Thyroid cancer underwent thyroidectomy	21	10 days	160 mg/day
	Ulcerative colitis	56	4 weeks	240 mg/day
	Pancreatic or biliary duct cancer	16	>9 months	200–400 mg/day
Theracurmin solution	Pancreatic or biliary duct cancer	16	>9 months	200–400 mg/day

Table 2.
List of some popular curcumin formulations that have been used in clinical studies in different disease conditions.

typically transient and occur over short time intervals. Therefore, it may not be necessary—or even ideal—for curcumin to achieve excessively high levels of systemic bioavailability. For instance, enhancing bioavailability by 2000-fold, as claimed to occur in the case of use in certain curcumin-piperine formulations, it could lead to indiscriminate distribution across all cell types, which might not be beneficial and could even introduce off-target effects. Instead, what is crucial is achieving a level of bioavailability that is sufficient for curcumin to reach the tumor microenvironment and remain in circulation long enough to exert its modulatory effects. A prolonged circulation time allows curcumin to engage with its relevant molecular targets within the tumor milieu, particularly those involved in maintaining immunosuppression. By modifying this immunosuppressive environment as well as modulating the intratumoral microbiota, curcumin can promote anti-tumor immune responses and facilitate the elimination of cancer cells. Thus, the therapeutic goal should not necessarily be indiscriminate maximal systemic exposure but rather optimized targeting with sustained local availability at the tumor site. Until robust head-to-head comparisons of different formulations are conducted, these questions remain unresolved. Additionally, despite the lack of preclinical data supporting curcumin's anticancer effects, relatively few high-quality clinical trials have been conducted. Encouragingly, the quality of studies has improved in recent years, with a growing number of trials reporting positive outcomes. However, for curcumin to gain widespread acceptance, it must be validated through well-powered, mechanistically sound investigations that incorporate international collaboration and standardized protocols.

The recent approaches have entailed different attempts to improve upon of curcumin's bioavailability by developing nanoformulations of curcumin, where the underlying idea was to achieve therapeutic concentrations of curcumin at the tissue site to exert its anticancer effects. The properties of nanocurcumin are influenced not only by its chemical composition but also by its physical attributes. These physicochemical characteristics contribute to its enhanced potency compared to conventional curcumin. Studies indicate that nanocurcumin's structural features improve its dissolution rate and bioavailability when administered orally. Tousif et al. prepared nanocurcumin by a modification of the nanoprecipitation method and without the use of any carrier particles to produce nanoparticles of pure curcumin having an average uniform size of ~200 nm. These curcumin nanoparticles exhibited greater bioavailability in mice and effectively reduced the hepatotoxicity induced by administration of anti-tubercular drugs to mice [64]. In another study, Dende et al. demonstrated the oral administration of a PLGA-based system containing 350 μg of curcumin led to a threefold increase in curcumin levels within brain tissue compared to an equivalent dose of free curcumin [65]. The reduction of curcumin particle size to the nanometer scale alters its properties, increasing its potency relative to native curcumin. The larger surface area of nanocurcumin makes it an effective pharmaceutical adjuvant, enabling penetration into organ systems that standard curcumin cannot access. A larger surface area also improves a drug's interaction with specific biological targets and its pharmacokinetic properties. Surface electrical charge is another crucial factor influencing nanocurcumin's behavior. Since curcumin has poor water solubility, conventional curcumin formulations tend to aggregate and become susceptible to opsonization. In contrast, nanocurcumin remains well-dispersed in aqueous solutions, avoiding aggregation due to its zeta potential. Nanoformulations of curcumin facilitate to improve the stability, and overall time that curcumin circulates and resides in the body. Additionally, nanocurcumin exhibits superior intracellular absorption, which is crucial for targeting curcumin in cancer cells. Delivering multiple cancer-fighting drugs together using nanoparticles is a promising approach for treating cancer. One method involves combining drugs that promote cancer cell death and block the formation of new blood vessels, which tumors need to grow. Zhang et al. created special pH-sensitive nanoparticles using a polymer to carry doxorubicin (Dox) and curcumin [66, 67]. These nanoparticles had a well-balanced drug ratio and efficient drug loading, and they released the drugs effectively in the acidic tumor environment. Compared to free drugs, these nanoparticles were better absorbed by liver cancer cells and endothelial cells. They caused significant cancer cell death by disrupting mitochondrial function and strongly inhibited blood vessel formation by blocking the VEGF signaling pathway. This combination of pro-apoptotic and antiangiogenic therapy within nanoparticles shows promise for treating liver cancer. Another emerging strategy is using metallic nanostructures to improve drug delivery. Kamble et al. studied curcumin-capped copper nanoparticles for their ability to slow blood vessel formation and cancer cell movement in breast cancer [68, 69]. However, these nanomaterials were less effective than free curcumin in reducing tumor growth and blocking angiogenesis. Similarly, Van der Vlies et al. developed curcumin-loaded polymeric nanoparticles using phenylboronic acid-containing structures [70]. These nanoparticles increased curcumin's stability and enabled controlled release. In a chicken embryo model, they significantly enhanced curcumin's ability to stop tumor growth and prevent new blood vessel formation [70]. In order to enhance curcumin's therapeutic impact, Zhu et al. prepared modified curcumin nanomaterials, which can selectively bind to transferrin receptors (TfR) overexpressed in lung cancer cells [71]. These nanostructures are also capable of regulating drug release in response to pH variations and oxidative stress. The dual-drug-loaded nanoparticles, incorporating curcumin and docetaxel (DTX), achieved drug-loading efficiencies of 7.82% and 6.48%, respectively. Even at higher concentrations (500 μg/mL), these nanomaterials maintained good biocompatibility. Most importantly, the combination therapy proved to be better compared to just docetaxel or conventional nanocarriers carrying either drug alone.

Additionally, nanomaterials were shown to modulate the tumor's immunosuppressive microenvironment, leading to enhanced tumor growth suppression. Another potent anti-cancer drug, camptothecin (CPT), has demonstrated efficacy against multiple cancers. However, its therapeutic potential in glioma is limited due to challenges in crossing the blood–brain barrier (BBB) and the highly immunosuppressive tumor environment. To overcome these barriers, researchers developed modified liposomes by the incorporation of tryptamine to facilitate the co-delivery of the drug along with curcumin [72]. The inclusion of tryptamine improved BBB penetration and enhanced the intracellular uptake of CPT, thereby inhibiting tumor cell proliferation. Additionally, the combination of curcumin and CPT helped counteract the PD-L1 upregulation caused by CPT, preventing T-cell inactivation and improving immune responses.

These findings provide a strong foundation for the potential use of curcumin-based nanoformultion in a combined approach for killing cancer cells, preventing angiogenesis, reducing immune suppression, enhancing anti-tumor immunity, and improving targeted drug delivery in cancer therapy. Nonetheless, the effectiveness of nanocurcumin for cancer treatment has been examined by only a limited number of clinical studies. While its properties provide a theoretical foundation for its therapeutic use, clinical evidence remains mixed, highlighting both promising trends and limitations. In one study on cisplatin-induced nephrotoxicity, nanocurcumin supplementation showed considerable efficacy. In the second study, however, it did not significantly prevent acute kidney injury, though a transient effect was observed after the first chemotherapy cycle. This suggests that either higher doses or prolonged administration may be necessary for meaningful nephroprotection.

For radiation-induced dermatitis in breast cancer patients, nanocurcumin supplementation was associated with reduced severity of skin reactions and improved pain management. However, statistical significance in overall severity reduction was only reached in the later stages of treatment, indicating a potential delayed therapeutic effect. Similarly, in bladder cancer patients, nanocurcumin supplementation showed a higher complete clinical response rate to chemotherapy, but the study lacked statistical power to confirm efficacy. This highlights the need for larger, more definitive trials to establish its therapeutic benefit. Regarding radiation-induced proctitis in prostate cancer patients, nanocurcumin did not show significant protection against radiation toxicity, though it was well-tolerated. The study's limited sample size may have affected the ability to detect potential benefits. The most compelling evidence for nanocurcumin's clinical application emerged in doxorubicin-induced cardiotoxicity in patients suffering from breast cancer. Nanocurcumin supplementation was correlated to the preservation of cardiac function, reducing the proportion of patients experiencing significant declines in left ventricular ejection fraction. This suggests a protective role against anthracycline-induced cardiac dysfunction. Taking insights from the few clinical trials involving the use of nanocurcumin in the treatment of cancer, we can understand that while the clinical benefits seemingly vary depending on the context, the most important emerging picture is that nanocurcumin appears to be safe and well-tolerated across multiple cancer settings. Certain studies are suggestive of a protective trend, particularly in reducing chemotherapy-related cardiotoxicity and radiation-induced skin reactions, but statistical significance in these studies is not consistently achieved, which may be a limitation of the study design and parameters in itself rather than a reflection of the efficacy of the molecule. It is therefore yet too early to discount nanocurcumin's efficacy in mitigating difficult-to-treat disorders based on the limited number of clinical studies that are available.

In summary of the points raised in the discussion, the following needs to be considered:

- Immunotherapy is going to cause severe adverse reactions due to cytokine storm, which can result in organ failure and neuro-toxicity. This has to be tackled if the immunotherapy has to be used routinely.

- The capability of nanocurcumin to enhance the cytotoxic capabilities of adoptive T-cell in a combination therapy should be explored further.

- The role of curcumin in the management of chronic pain arising due to inflammatory responses, nerve compression, and adverse effects of conventional therapies needs to be investigated.

- The curcumin formulations used in clinical trials have to be standardized in terms of absorption distribution metabolism excretion (ADME) characteristics so that different formulations can be compared with each other.

6. Conclusion

There is a need to conduct large-scale, placebo-controlled, double-blind, long-term clinical trials to establish the efficacy and safety profile of well-characterized curcumin nanoformulation using patients from various cancer types. For monitoring the role of curcumin, suitable biomarkers have to be analyzed at different stages of treatment. Oral delivery of nanocurcumin will modulate gut microbiome, which will have to be analyzed along with how it affects the tumor microbiota. The potential of nanocurcumin as an agent for palliative care for cancer patients needs to be investigated.

Author details

Sitabja Mukherjee and Santosh K. Kar*
Polyfeenolix Research Laboratory, Biotechnology Incubator, KIIT University, Bhubaneswar, Odisha, India

*Address all correspondence to: santoshkar1946@gmail.com

References

[1] Coley WB. The treatment of malignant tumors by repeated inoculations of erysipelas. With a report of ten original cases. 1893. Clinical Orthopaedics and Related Research. 1991;**262**:3-11

[2] Chen J, Gao L, Wu X, Fan Y, Liu M, Peng L, et al. BCG- induced trained immunity: History, mechanisms and potential applications. Journal of Translational Medicine. 2023;**21**(1):106. DOI: 10.1186/s12967-023-03944-8

[3] Jiang S, Redelman-Sidi G. BCG in bladder cancer immunotherapy. Cancers (Basel). 2022;**14**(13):3073. DOI: 10.3390/cancers14133073

[4] Gupta KH, Nowicki C, Giurini EF, Marzo AL, Zloza A. Bacterial-based cancer therapy (BBCT): Recent advances, current challenges, and future prospects for cancer immunotherapy. Vaccines (Basel). 2021;**9**(12):1497. DOI: 10.3390/vaccines9121497

[5] Zahavi D, Weiner L. Monoclonal antibodies in cancer therapy. Antibodies (Basel). 2020;**9**(3):34. DOI: 10.3390/antib9030034

[6] Wang J, Zhou K, Zhu H, Wei F, Ma S, Kan Y, et al. Current status and progress of the development of prostate cancer vaccines. Journal of Cancer. 2023;**14**(5): 835-842. DOI: 10.7150/jca.80803

[7] Sharma P, Goswami S, Raychaudhuri D, Siddiqui BA, Singh P, Nagarajan A, et al. Immune checkpoint therapy-current perspectives and future directions. Cell. 2023;**186**(8):1652-1669. DOI: 10.1016/j.cell.2023.03.006

[8] Wojtukiewicz MZ, Rek MM, Karpowicz K, Górska M, Polityńska B, Wojtukiewicz AM, et al. Inhibitors of immune checkpoints-PD-1, PD-L1, CTLA-4-new opportunities for cancer patients and a new challenge for internists and general practitioners. Cancer Metastasis Reviews. 2021;**40**(3): 949-982. DOI: 10.1007/s10555-021-09976-0

[9] Sterner RC, Sterner RM. CAR-T cell therapy: Current limitations and potential strategies. Blood Cancer Journal. 2021;**11**(4):69. DOI: 10.1038/s41408-021-00459-7

[10] Nguyen HH, Bui KC, Nguyen TML, Pham C, Nham TPL, Ngo TH, et al. The safety of CAR-T cells and PD-1 antibody combination on an experimental model. Biochemical and Biophysical Research Communications. 2023;**649**:25-31. DOI: 10.1016/j.bbrc.2023.01.096

[11] Vivier E, Rebuffet L, Narni-Mancinelli E, Cornen S, Igarashi RY, Fantin VR. Natural killer cell therapies. Nature. 2024;**626**(8000):727-736. DOI: 10.1038/s41586-023- 06945-1

[12] Mantovani A, Allavena P, Marchesi F, Garlanda C. Macrophages as tools and targets in cancer therapy. Nature Reviews. Drug Discovery. 2022; **21**(11):799-820. DOI: 10.1038/s41573-022-00520-5

[13] Pittet MJ, Di Pilato M, Garris C, Mempel TR. Dendritic cells as shepherds of T cell immunity in cancer. Immunity. 2023;**56**(10):2218-2230. DOI: 10.1016/j.immuni.2023.08.014

[14] Yang D, Liu J, Qian H, Zhuang Q. Cancer-associated fibroblasts: From basic science to anticancer therapy. Experimental and Molecular Medicine. 2023;**55**(7):1322-1332. DOI: 10.1038/s12276- 023-01013-0

[15] Xu R, Zhou X, Wang S, Trinkle C. Tumor organoid models in precision medicine and investigating cancer-stromal interactions. Pharmacology and Therapeutics. 2021;**218**:107668. DOI: 10.1016/j.pharmthera.2020.107668

[16] Pelletier V. The Journal de Pharmacie Clinique. 1815;**I**:289

[17] Milobedzka J, Kostanecki S, Lampe V. Zur Kenntnis des Curcumins. Berichte der Deutschen Chemischen Gesellschaft. 1910;**43**:2163-2170

[18] Lampe V, Milobedzka J. Studien uber Curcumin. Berichte der Deutschen Chemischen Gesellschaft. 1913;**46**: 2235-2240. DOI: 10.1002/cber.191304602149

[19] Srinivasan KR. A chromatographic study of the curcuminoids in Curcuma longa, L. The Journal of Pharmacy and Pharmacology. 1953;**5**:448-457. DOI: 10.1111/j.2042-7158.1953.tb14007.x

[20] Gasbarri C, Angelini G. Cyclocurcumin as promising bioactive natural compound: An overview. Molecules. 2024;**29**(7):1451. DOI: 10.3390/molecules29071451

[21] Cardoso BD, Rodrigues ARO, Almeida BG, Amorim CO, Amaral VS, Castanheira EMS, et al. Stealth magnetoliposomes based on calcium-substituted magnesium ferrite nanoparticles for curcumin transport and release. International Journal of Molecular Sciences. 2020;**21**(10):3641. DOI: 10.3390/ijms21103641

[22] Shoba G, Joy D, Joseph T, Majeed M, Rajendran R, Srinivas PS. Influence of piperine on the pharmacokinetics of curcumin in animals and human volunteers. Planta Medica. 1998;**64**(4): 353-356. DOI: 10.1055/s-2006-957450

[23] Sharma RA, Euden SA, Platton SL, Cooke DN, Shafayat A, Hewitt HR, et al. Phase I clinical trial of oral curcumin: Biomarkers of systemic activity and compliance. Clinical Cancer Research. 2004;**10**(20):6847-6854. DOI: 10.1158/1078-0432.CCR-04-0744

[24] Yang KY, Lin LC, Tseng TY, Wang SC, Tsai TH. Oral bioavailability of curcumin in rat and the herbal analysis from Curcuma longa by LC-MS/MS. Journal of Chromatography B: Analytical Technologies in the Biomedical and Life Sciences. 2007;**853** (1–2):183-189. DOI: 10.1016/j.jchromb.2007.03.010

[25] Garcea G, Berry DP, Jones DJ, Singh R, Dennison AR, Farmer PB, et al. Detection of curcumin and its metabolites in hepatic tissue and portal blood of patients following oral administration. British Journal of Cancer. 2005;**93**(8):963-967. DOI: 10.1038/sj.bjc.6601623

[26] Roshan Z, Haddadi-Asl V, Ahmadi H, Moussaei M. Curcumin-encapsulated poly(lactic-co-glycolic acid) nanoparticles: A comparison of drug release kinetics from particles prepared via electrospray and nanoprecipitation. Macromolecular Materials and Engineering. 2024;**309**(7): 2400040. DOI: 10.1002/mame.202400040

[27] Sanoj Rejinold N, Sreerekha PR, Chennazhi KP, Nair SV, Jayakumar R. Biocompatible, biodegradable and thermo-sensitive chitosan-g-poly (N-isopropylacrylamide) nanocarrier for curcumin drug delivery. International Journal of Biological Macromolecules. 2011;**49**(2):161-172. DOI: 10.1016/j.ijbiomac.2011.04.008

[28] Wang Y, Zhang K, Qin M, Ding F, Xu Q, Zhang J, et al. Production of

curcumin- loaded silk fibroin nanoparticles for cancer therapy. Nanomaterials (Basel). 2018;**8**(2):126. DOI: 10.3390/nano8020126

[29] Sanoj Rejinold N, Sreerekha PR, Chennazhi KP, Nair SV, Jayakumar R. Biocompatible, biodegradable and thermo-sensitive chitosan-g-poly (N-isopropylacrylamide) nanocarrier for curcumin drug delivery. International Journal of Biological Macromolecules. 2011;**49**(2):161-172. DOI: 10.1016/j.ijbiomac.2011.04.008

[30] Bhawana BRK, Buttar HS, Jain VK, Jain N. Curcumin nanoparticles: Preparation, characterization, and antimicrobial study. Journal of Agricultural and Food Chemistry. 2011; **59**(5):2056-2061. DOI: 10.1021/jf104402t

[31] Martínez Rivas CJ, Tarhini M, Badri W, Miladi K, Greige-Gerges H, Nazari QA, et al. Nanoprecipitation process: From encapsulation to drug delivery. International Journal of Pharmaceutics. 2017;**532**(1):66-81. DOI: 10.1016/j.ijpharm.2017.08.064

[32] Jenjob R, Phakkeeree T, Seidi F, Theerasilp M, Crespy D. Emulsion techniques for the production of pharmacological nanoparticles. Macromolecular Bioscience. 2019;**19**(6): e1900063. DOI: 10.1002/mabi.201900063

[33] Subramani T, Ganapathyswamy H. An overview of liposomal nano-encapsulation techniques and its applications in food and nutraceutical. Journal of Food Science and Technology. 2020;**57**(10):3545-3555. DOI: 10.1007/s13197-020-04360-2

[34] Gupta T, Singh J, Kaur S, Sandhu S, Singh G, Kaur IP. Enhancing bioavailability and stability of curcumin using solid lipid nanoparticles (CLEN): A covenant for its effectiveness. Frontiers in Bioengineering and Biotechnology. 2020;**8**:879. DOI: 10.3389/fbioe.2020.00879

[35] Feltrin FDS, Agner T, Sayer C, Lona LMF. Curcumin encapsulation in functional PLGA nanoparticles: A promising strategy for cancer therapies. Advances in Colloid and Interface Science. 2022;**300**:102582. DOI: 10.1016/j.cis.2021.102582

[36] Kumbhar S, Khairate R, Bhatia M, Choudhari P, Gaikwad V. Evaluation of curcumin- loaded chitosan nanoparticles for wound healing activity. ADMET DMPK. 2023;**11**(4):601-613. DOI: 10.5599/admet.1897

[37] Preeti SS, Malik R, Bhatia S, Al Harrasi A, Rani C, Saharan R, et al. Nanoemulsion: An emerging novel technology for improving the bioavailability of drugs. Scientifica (Cairo). 2023;**2023**:6640103. DOI: 10.1155/2023/6640103

[38] Ghezzi M, Pescina S, Padula C, Santi P, Del Favero E, Cantù L, et al. Polymeric micelles in drug delivery: An insight of the techniques for their characterization and assessment in biorelevant conditions. Journal of Controlled Release. 2021;**332**:312-336. DOI: 10.1016/j.jconrel.2021.02.031

[39] Yang X, Li Z, Wang N, Li L, Song L, He T, et al. Curcumin-encapsulated polymeric micelles suppress the development of colon cancer in vitro and in vivo. Scientific Reports. 2015;**5**:10322. DOI: 10.1038/srep10322

[40] Dokania S, Joshi AK. Self-microemulsifying drug delivery system (SMEDDS)– challenges and road ahead. Drug Delivery. 2015;**22**(6):675-690. DOI: 10.3109/10717544.2014.896058

[41] Wang Y, Li Z, Fayu S, Li F, Wang W. Preparation of curcumin submicron particles by supercritical antisolvent method with external adjustable annular gap nozzle. Scientific Reports. 2025;**15**(1):3312. DOI: 10.1038/s41598-025-87787-x

[42] Lin P, Gu H, Zhuang X, Wang F, Hu X. Controlled release of curcumin and hypocrellin a from ElectrospunPoly (l-lactic acid)/silk fibroin nanofibers for enhanced cancer cell inhibition. ACS Applied Bio Materials. 2024;**7**(8): 5423-5436. DOI: 10.1021/acsabm.4c00582

[43] Rai DB, Medicherla K, Pooja D, Kulhari H. Dendrimer-mediated delivery of anticancer drugs for colon cancer treatment. Pharmaceutics. 2023;**15**(3): 801. DOI: 10.3390/pharmaceutics15030801

[44] Mehrab H, Sharifi M, Akhavan A, Aarabi MH, Mansourian M, Mosavi E, et al. Curcumin supplementation prevents cisplatin-induced nephrotoxicity: A randomized, double-blinded, and placebo-controlled trial. Research in Pharmaceutical Sciences. 2023;**18**(6):648-662. DOI: 10.4103/1735-5362.389952

[45] Hosseini S, Rahsepar S, Naghipour S, Elyasi S. Is oral nano-curcumin formulation a safe and effective measure for preventing cisplatin-induced nephrotoxicity in cancer patients? Anti-Cancer Drugs. 2024;**35**(9):859-866. DOI: 10.1097/CAD.0000000000001639

[46] Talakesh T, Tabatabaee N, Atoof F, Aliasgharzadeh A, Sarvizade M, Farhood B, et al. Effect of Nano-curcumin on radiotherapy-induced skin reaction in breast cancer patients: A randomized, triple-blind, placebo-controlled trial. Current Radiopharmaceuticals. 2022;**15**(4): 332-340. DOI: 10.2174/1874471015666220623104316

[47] Sandoughdaran S, Razzaghdoust A, Tabibi A, Basiri A, Simforoosh N, Mofid B. Randomized, double-blind pilot study of Nanocurcumin in bladder cancer patients receiving induction chemotherapy. Urology Journal. 2021; **18**(3):295-300. DOI: 10.22037/uj.v0i0.5719

[48] Saadipoor A, Razzaghdoust A, Simforoosh N, Mahdavi A, Bakhshandeh M, Moghadam M, et al. Randomized, double-blind, placebo-controlled phase II trial of nanocurcumin in prostate cancer patients undergoing radiotherapy. Phytotherapy Research. 2019;**33**(2):370-378. DOI: 10.1002/ptr.6230

[49] Tohidi M, Allahyari A, Ataei Azimi S, Alimi H, Elyasi S, Qoorchi Moheb Seraj F, et al. The protective effect of nano curcumin supplementation on doxorubicin induced cardiotoxicity in breast cancer patients; a randomized, double- blind clinical trial. Journal of Oncology Pharmacy Practice. 2024: 10781552241277958. DOI: 10.1177/10781552241277958 [Online ahead of print]

[50] Shah S, Rath H, Sharma G, Senapati SN, Mishra E. Effectiveness of curcumin mouthwash on radiation-induced oral mucositis among head and neck cancer patients: A triple-blind, pilot randomised controlled trial. Indian Journal of Dental Research. 2020;**31**(5): 718-727. DOI: 10.4103/ijdr.IJDR_822_18

[51] Nejman D, Livyatan I, Fuks G, Gavert N, Zwang Y, Geller LT, et al. The human tumor microbiome is composed of tumor type-specific intracellular bacteria. Science. 2020;**368**(6494): 973-980. DOI: 10.1126/science.aay9189

[52] Ge Y, Wang X, Guo Y, Yan J, Abuduwaili A, Aximujiang K, et al. Gut microbiota influence tumor development and Alter interactions with the human immune system. Journal of Experimental and Clinical Cancer Research. 2021;**40**(1):42. DOI: 10.1186/s13046-021-01845-6. Erratum in: J Exp Clin Cancer Res. 2021;40(1):334. doi: 10.1186/s13046-021-02131-1

[53] Zhu J, He L. The modulatory effects of curcumin on the gut microbiota: A potential strategy for disease treatment and health promotion. Microorganisms. 2024;**12**(4):642. DOI: 10.3390/microorganisms12040642

[54] Yang L, Wang Q, He L, Sun X. The critical role of tumor microbiome in cancer immunotherapy. Cancer Biology and Therapy. 2024;**25**(1):2301801. DOI: 10.1080/15384047.2024.2301801

[55] Zheng D, Liwinski T, Elinav E. Interaction between microbiota and immunity in health and disease. Cell Research. 2020;**30**:492-506. DOI: 10.1038/s41422-020-0332-7

[56] Cao Y, Xia H, Tan X, Shi C, Ma Y, Meng D, et al. Intratumoural microbiota: A new frontier in cancer development and therapy. Signal Transduction and Targeted Therapy. 2024;**9**(1):15

[57] Yousefi Y, Baines KJ, Maleki VS. Microbiome bacterial influencers of host immunity and response to immunotherapy. Cell Reports Medicine. 2024;**5**(4):101487

[58] Li C, Jiang P, Wei S, Xu X, Wang J. Regulatory T cells in tumor microenvironment: New mechanisms, potential therapeutic strategies and future prospects. Molecular Cancer. 2020;**19**(1):116

[59] Zhu C, Zhao Y, He J, Zhao H, Ni L, Cheng X, et al. TIL-derived CAR T cells improve immune cell infiltration and survival in the treatment of CD19-humanized mouse colorectal cancer. Cancers (Basel). 2023;**15**(23):5567

[60] Wang Y, Lu J, Jiang B, Guo J. The roles of curcumin in regulating the tumor immunosuppressive microenvironment. Oncology Letters. 2020;**19**(4):3059-3070. DOI: 10.3892/ol.2020.11437

[61] Chang YF, Chuang HY, Hsu CH, Liu RS, Gambhir SS, Hwang JJ. Immunomodulation of curcumin on adoptive therapy with T cell functional imaging in mice. Cancer Prevention Research (Philadelphia, Pa.). 2012;**5**(3): 444-452. DOI: 10.1158/1940- 6207. CAPR-11-0308

[62] Basu P, Maier C. Basu A, Effects of curcumin and its different formulations in preclinical and clinical studies of peripheral neuropathic and postoperative pain: A comprehensive review. International Journal of Molecular Sciences. 2021;**22**(9):4666. DOI: 10.3390/ijms22094666

[63] Hegde M, Girisa S, BharathwajChetty B, Vishwa R, Kunnumakkara AB. Curcumin formulations for better bioavailability: What we learned from clinical trials thus far? ACS Omega. 2023;**8**(12): 10713-10746

[64] Tousif S, Singh DK, Mukherjee S, Ahmad S, Arya R, Nanda R, et al. Nanoparticle-formulated curcumin prevents Posttherapeutic disease reactivation and reinfection with *mycobacterium tuberculosis* following isoniazid therapy. Frontiers in Immunology. 2017;**8**:739. DOI: 10.3389/fimmu.2017.00739

[65] Dende C, Meena J, Nagarajan P, Nagaraj VA, Panda AK, Padmanaban G.

Nanocurcumin is superior to native curcumin in preventing degenerative changes in experimental cerebral malaria. Scientific Reports. 2017;7(1): 10062. DOI: 10.1038/s41598-017-10672-9

[66] Zhang Y, Yang C, Wang W, Liu J, Liu Q, Huang F, et al. Co-delivery of doxorubicin and curcumin by pH-sensitive prodrug nanoparticle for combination therapy of cancer. Scientific Reports. 2016;**6**:21225. DOI: 10.1038/srep21225

[67] Zhang J, Li J, Shi Z, Yang Y, Xie X, Lee SM, et al. pH- sensitive polymeric nanoparticles for co-delivery of doxorubicin and curcumin to treat cancer via enhanced pro-apoptotic and anti-angiogenic activities. Acta Biomaterialia. 2017;**58**:349-364. DOI: 10.1016/j.actbio.2017.04.029

[68] Kamble S, Utage B, Mogle P, Kamble R, Hese S, Dawane B, et al. Evaluation of curcumin capped copper nanoparticles as possible inhibitors of human breast cancer cells and angiogenesis: A comparative study with native curcumin. AAPS PharmSciTech. 2016;**17**(5):1030-1041. DOI: 10.1208/s12249-015-0435-5

[69] der Vlies AJ, Morisaki M, Neng HI, Hansen EM, Hasegawa U. Framboidal nanoparticles containing a curcumin-phenylboronic acid complex with antiangiogenic and anticancer activities. Bioconjugate Chemistry. 2019;**30**(3): 861-870. DOI: 10.1021/acs.bioconjchem.9b00006

[70] Zhu X, Yu Z, Feng L, Deng L, Fang Z, Liu Z, et al. Chitosan-based nanoparticle co-delivery of docetaxel and curcumin ameliorates anti- tumor chemoimmunotherapy in lung cancer. Carbohydrate Polymers. 2021;**268**: 118237. DOI: 10.1016/j.carbpol.2021.118237

[71] Wang Z, Wang X, Yu H, Chen M. Glioma-targeted multifunctional nanoparticles to co-deliver camptothecin and curcumin for enhanced chemo-immunotherapy. Biomaterials Science. 2022;**10**(5):1292-1303. DOI: 10.1039/d1bm01987b

[72] Wang Z, Wang X, Yu H, Chen M. Glioma-targeted multifunctional nanoparticles to co-deliver camptothecin and curcumin for enhanced chemo-immunotherapy. Biomaterials Science. 2022;**10**(5):1292-1303. DOI: 10.1039/d1bm01987b